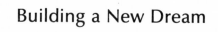

Building a New Dream

Building a New Dream

A Family Guide to Coping with Chronic Illness and Disability

◆ —————————————— ◆

Janet R. Maurer, M.D.
Patricia D. Strasberg, Ed.D.

Addison-Wesley Publishing Company, Inc.
Reading, Massachusetts   Menlo Park, California   New York
Don Mills, Ontario   Wokingham, England   Amsterdam   Bonn
Sydney   Singapore   Tokyo   Madrid   San Juan

Many of the designations used by manufacturers and sellers to distinguish their products are claimed as trademarks. Where those designations appear in this book and Addison-Wesley was aware of a trademark claim, the designations have been printed in initial capital letters (e.g., Pepsi).

Library of Congress Cataloging-in-Publication Data

Maurer, Janet R.
  Building a new dream.

  Bibliography: p.
  Includes index.
    1. Chronic diseases—Psychological aspects—Handbooks,
manuals, etc.   2. Chronic diseases—Social aspects—
Handbooks, manuals, etc.   I. Strasberg, Patricia D.
II. Title.
RC108.M38   1989   362.1'042   89-6994
ISBN 0-201-09364-2
ISBN 0-201-55098-9 (pbk.)

Cover design by Copenhaver Cumpston
Text design by Joyce C. Weston
Set in 11 point Times Roman by DEKR Corporation, Woburn, MA

ABCDEFG-DO-93210
First paperback printing, June 1990

Contents

Where to Find Illnesses of Particular Interest to You

We have written this book to cover situations that might be encountered by persons facing any long-term illness, and we feel that any family will find something of personal interest in each chapter. Adjustment to some illnesses, however, may be hampered by particular difficulties. The following is a list of common types of illness or disability, followed by chapters that are especially relevant to those problems.

AIDS
Section 1: Chapters 2, 4, 5
Section 2: Chapters 6, 7, 9, 10, 13
Section 3: Chapters 14, 16

Alzheimer's Disease (and Other Dementing Diseases)
Section 1: Chapters 2, 5
Section 2: Chapters 6, 9, 10
Section 3: Chapter 16

Amputation and Congenital Deformities
Section 1: Chapters 2, 5
Section 2: Chapters 6, 7, 8, 11, 12
Section 3: All chapters

Arthritis
Section 1: Chapters 2, 3, 5
Section 2: Chapters 6, 7, 11
Section 3: All chapters

Asthma
Section 1: Chapters 1, 2, 4
Section 2: Chapters 6, 8, 10, 13
Section 3: All chapters

Blindness (Retinitis Pigmentosa, Glaucoma, etc.)
Section 1: Chapters 1, 3, 5
Section 2: Chapters 6, 7, 11, 12
Section 3: All chapters

Cancer
Section 1: All chapters
Section 2: Chapters 6, 7, 8, 11, 12, 13
Section 3: Chapters 14, 16

Cerebral Palsy
Section 1: Chapters 2, 5
Section 2: Chapters 6, 7, 11, 12
Section 3: Chapters 14, 16

Chronic Lung Disease (Emphysema, Bronchitis, Interstitial Fibrosis)
Section 1: Chapters 1, 2, 4, 5
Section 2: Chapters 7, 8, 10, 11, 12, 13
Section 3: All chapters

Colitis (See Inflammatory Bowel Disease)

Collagen Vascular Disease (Systemic Lupus Erythematosus, Scleroderma, Myositis, Mixed Connective Tissue Disease, etc.)
Section 1: Chapters 1, 2, 3, 5
Section 2: Chapters 6, 7, 9, 10, 11
Section 3: All chapters

Cystic Fibrosis
Section 1: Chapters 4, 5
Section 2: Chapters 6, 7, 10, 13
Section 3: Chapters 14, 16

Diabetes Mellitus
Section 1: Chapters 1, 2, 3, 5
Section 2: Chapters 6, 7, 10, 11, 12
Section 3: All chapters

Epilepsy (See Seizure Disorders.)

Heart Disease
Section 1: All chapters
Section 2: Chapters 6, 7, 8, 10, 12, 13
Section 3: All chapters

Hereditary Disease (Refer to organs affected. For example, for Huntington's Disease, look under Neurologic Disorders.) Of particular importance to all persons with these illnesses is
Section 1: Chapter 1.

Hypertension
Section 1: Chapters 1, 2
Section 2: Chapters 6, 12
Section 3: Chapters 14, 17

Inflammatory Bowel Disease (Ileitis, Colitis, Crohn's, etc.)
Section 1: Chapters 1, 2, 5
Section 2: Chapters 6, 7, 11, 12
Section 3: All chapters

Kidney Disease
Section 1: Chapters 2, 4, 5
Section 2: Chapters 6, 7, 9, 10, 12, 13
Section 3: All chapters

Liver Disease
Section 1: Chapters 1, 4, 5
Section 2: Chapters 6, 7, 10, 11
Section 3: Chapters 14, 15, 17

Multiple Sclerosis (and Similar Diseases)
Section 1: Chapters 1, 2, 4, 5
Section 2: Chapters 6, 7, 8, 10, 11, 12
Section 3: All chapters

Neurologic Disorders (Parkinson's Disease, Huntington's Disease, Muscular Dystrophy,

ALS, Guillain-Barré Syndrome, Sequelae of Head Trauma, etc.)
Section 1: Chapters 1, 2, 4, 5
Section 2: All chapters
Section 3: All chapters

Organ Transplant
Section 1: Chapters 2, 3, 4
Section 2: All chapters
Section 3: All chapters

Pain
Section 1: Chapters 1, 2, 4, 5
Section 2: Chapters 6, 7, 9, 10, 12
Section 3: Chapters 15, 16

Seizure Disorders (Epilepsy, etc.)
Section 1: Chapters 1, 2, 4
Section 2: Chapters 6, 8, 9, 10, 11, 13
Section 3: Chapters 14, 15, 17

Spinal Cord Injury (Fixed Paralysis Due to Accident or Illness)
Section 1: Chapters 2, 3, 4, 5
Section 2: Chapters 6, 7, 8, 10, 11, 12
Section 3: All chapters

Stroke
Section 1: Chapters 2, 3, 4, 5
Section 2: All chapters
Section 3: All chapters

Skin Disorders
Section 1: Chapter 1
Section 2: Chapters 6, 7, 9, 12
Section 3: Chapters 15, 16

Ulcer Disease
Section 1: Chapters 1, 2
Section 2: Chapters 7, 8
Section 3: Chapters 14, 15, 17

Introduction

Is your family trying to cope with the ongoing physical illness or physical disability of one of its members? You. are not alone. The emotional and social pressures that your family is experiencing are similar to those felt by millions of other families dealing with chronic illness. And, like you, they probably had little forewarning and were ill prepared for the dramatic impact a single illness would have on the lives of all family members.

Many advances have been made in medicine, yet few cures have been found for many of the diseases that affect adults. The impact of medical research has been in the designing of treatments and medication that decrease symptoms. Yet, the disease often is still present, and the patient and family must "learn to live with it." That often made statement is not so easy to carry out, since even with therapy, most ongoing illnesses cause gradual loss of function and increasing limitations in all aspects of the person's life.

Depending on the phase of a person's life in which it occurs, the shattering impact of illness may be equally pervasive but quite different. A young man stricken with multiple sclerosis may be distraught over the inability to support his family or teach his children to play basketball; a person nearing retirement may see the dreams of world travel he has planned for thirty-five years disappear with a paralyzing stroke.

Complicating those losses is an unwritten rule commanding silence. It has been traditional in our culture to be ashamed of illness, to try to hide it and keep "our little secret." This makes recognizing, let alone coping, with the many facets of chronic illness that much more difficult. With poor communication, the illness becomes a festering sore—a source of continuing but un-addressed irritation that eventually erodes the family structure.

The family suffers with the ill person, often not cognizant of the pervasive effect of the illness. Financial difficulties arise if a person cannot work or has high medical bills, and these compound the stress; interpersonal and social relationships are neglected, and families can fall apart almost before they realize what is happening. Worse, this is all at a time when the members most need each other's support.

Sometimes family members feel so much tension or anger or frustration, they wonder if they are going crazy. The mental anguish accompanying physical illness is often so severe that patients and families need outside counseling to help them cope. Yet, again, our culture has traditionally taught us that we should solve these problems ourselves. We have not been allowed the option of asking for outside help in coping with emotional devastation!

This book is designed to help families recognize emotional and social stress, and then to offer suggestions for dealing with these stresses. It is for families who find themselves fighting a long-term physical illness or injury of any kind—kidney failure, diabetes, paralysis, other neurologic diseases, AIDS, heart disease, multiple sclerosis, colitis, cancer, emphysema, ulcers, liver cirrhosis, chronic back pain, etc. It really does not matter what organ system is involved; many of the nonmedical issues that families must confront are common to all.

We have chosen a vignette-comment format to do this. That is, we will describe a typical social or family encounter and follow it by an explanation of how the family might recognize and deal with problems and issues illustrated by the vignette. Though the vignettes do not represent any specific families and any name similarities to real situations are purely coincidental, they do draw from our combined experiences. Most families will likely identify with a number of the vignette illustrations, even if they are coping with a different physical illness, as the situations presented are very common regardless of the specific illness that has occurred. The book has three main sections. The first is a guide to learning about the illness and working with health professionals. A section on handling medical crises is also included. We feel that a good understanding of the disease and its probable course, as well as medication effects and side effects, is essential. Informed patients find coping with nonmedical issues less difficult and can more readily call upon the professional services that might improve their lives.

The second section centers on the emotional trauma that is likely to occur to the individual and to the family. The third section deals with the social impact of illness. There is necessarily some carryover between these sections, and we have tried to emphasize the nuclear interpersonal relationships in Section 2. In both sections, each chapter will contain vignettes covering individuals and families both in their young adult or prime family and earning years, as well as persons who are in another life phase near retirement. When one's sex or the fact that one might be a single person or single parent has a particular impact on the type of problem encountered, appropriate vignettes will be presented.

It is our hope that this book will help families recognize problems in coping and stimulate improved communications. Ultimately, our goal is to encourage individual members not to withdraw from each other when what they need most is mutual support. We want to help them recognize the situations wherein they need help in coping, and urge them in those cases to seek out outside help for counseling. We will suggest ways in which to do this.

And finally, we believe that these nonphysical issues accompanying chronic physical illnesses can be largely overcome and that most people can successfully and happily adapt to a new lifestyle. They can "learn to live with it" for many years.

ONE

Working with Health Professionals in the Community

◆ ——————————— ◆

CHAPTER 1

Learning All about Your Illness

The first step to successfully coping with an illness is to obtain enough information to understand the potential impact of the problem on all facets of your life—personal, work, family, and social.

Learning about the illness may be easier for those people who are naturally gregarious and cope by gaining information and asking questions. However, most of us are shy and find the prospect of illness not only frightening but also threatening. We wish we could just forget about it, and in the back of our minds hope against hope that it will just go away. Unfortunately that does not often happen; even worse, those of us who try to cope by ignoring the illness have more difficulty in approaching the doctor to get information. We are often intimidated by the doctor's knowledge or are afraid he/she might reveal something terrible about what will happen in the future as the illness gets worse. Many of us are also intimidated because we really do not know how to go about asking the right questions to get the most useful information.

Because a person's understanding of his illness or injury is so important to his ultimate success in coping with all aspects of it, this first chapter offers some guidelines about the most effective ways to get information from the doctor, what information is important to have, and how to use the information you get. We also talk about some general guidelines to follow in establishing a good doctor-patient relationship, in the belief that this will lessen the feelings of intimidation that many patients (even other doctors) feel when discussing such personal problems with their physicians.

The final section addresses some of the feelings and needs peculiar to the illnesses that go on for many months or years. In such situations, the relationships between the doctor and the patient can be characterized by very intense feelings and different expectations. Nonphysician resources for persons and families suffering chronic illness are further explored in Chapter 5.

◆ Mike walked into Dr. Mill's office feeling great. He had applied for life insurance and he had to have a physical to get it approved. He was forty-two but felt thirty, exercised every day, and was in great shape. The blow came as he sat in the doctor's office after the exam. "We have a little problem here," he remembered him saying, "your blood pressure is quite high and we'll have to watch it." As he walked home, Mike tried to remember what else had been said, but he could not recall any of it—yet he had spent a good twenty minutes talking to the doctor.

It is common to think of ourselves as invulnerable to illness or serious injury and even hope that if we live right or exercise and eat properly, it will never happen to us. In a sense, this is a means of self-preservation because our cultural attitudes very much discriminate against the sick person. In our society, sick people are considered different, outsiders, and a group to which we do not wish to belong. Sick people or people with serious permanent injuries find themselves without jobs and dropped from their usual social circles. Thus, to be ill is a real insult to one's integrity and a constant reminder of one's mortality. Even if an illness can be controlled with medication or other treatment, being tied to pills is a constant reminder of the presence of the intruding problem.

Thus it is not surprising that when hit with an unexpected diagnosis, the shock is such that we remember little of what has been said to us in the initial visit. In coping successfully with your new diagnosis, cardinal rule number one is to remember to schedule a follow-up appointment soon after the initial appointment, for the sole purpose of discussing the new diagnosis and its potential impact on your life. It is best to let several days elapse (if this is medically possible) to allow yourself time to adjust to the idea of having an ongoing medical condition.

In the example above, Mike was totally surprised by his diagnosis because he felt well when he visited the doctor. When a person visits the doctor, complaining of some symptoms, in the back of his mind he may suspect he has a serious illness. Yet even in this situation, most of us hope we are wrong, and when given bad news remember very little of the conversation. These situations require follow-up visits to discuss the diagnosis and gain information as well.

◆ Mike's initial shock at learning he likely had a chronic medical problem gradually wore off over the next few days and was replaced by concern about the likely future. He realized that there were a lot of things he did not know about high blood pressure and his head was filled with questions. Could he do something to lower the pressure? Was he in any danger? His mind was skipping around, and he was confused and frightened. His work began to suffer because of his preoccupation with his health.

In fact, Mike's doctor had discussed these questions and many others during the twenty-minute office visit; but as a normal human reaction is to block out unpleasant news, Mike heard and remembered very little. For his follow-up visit two weeks later, Mike decided to prepare himself so that he would get the information that he wanted about his high blood pressure. He could then begin to adjust positively to the problem. He would need to get the questions answered in such a way that he could remember the information and use it to change his life-style or make whatever adaptations were necessary to reduce future complications or other problems.

This is a very successful attitude in beginning to cope with a new illness. To get the best and most useful information, it is helpful to follow the basic principles listed here. These suggestions will help organize your thoughts and your visit with the doctor. He/she will appreciate the effort you have put into preparing for your visit, and the time can be very productive for both of you.

1. Think about the types of information you need ahead of time. Think about the type of questions, especially those particularly relevant to your life-style, for which you will need answers (see Chapter 2, Adjusting to Medication and Other Therapy). Write them down in order of priority and category. For example, questions about "cause of illness" should all be asked together; questions about "treatment" should be grouped together. Skipping back and forth from one aspect of the illness to another will be confusing, and your memory of the information given will be less accurate than if you use an organized approach. Also, it is much easier for the doctor to maintain a train of thought if he/she does not have to skip back and forth from area to area, and you are likely to get more overall information.

2. Display interest. Doctors like to talk about their work just as anyone does. If you show an interest in learning about the illness, you will probably have no difficulty getting more information than you want!

3. Don't be embarrassed to ask for clarification. Sometimes doctors are so used to speaking in the technical terms of the profession that they do not realize they are using words you do not understand. Far from thinking you are dumb for not understanding them, they would appreciate your reminding them that they are speaking over your head. The purpose of an information session is just that; if the information is unintelligible, you will be frustrated and angry, but if you do not speak up, the doctor will not even know there is a miscommunication. This sort of unnecessary, unresolved issue is often the basis of a destroyed doctor-patient relationship that could otherwise be very good.

Sometimes it may be necessary to ask the doctor to draw a picture of an injury or a disease process to help you understand the concept of the problem. It is easier for most of us to visualize something if it can be illustrated for us. Once you have thought over the information given, you might find that you do not completely understand the illness. In this case, you may at future visits need to ask for a repeat explanation or an alternate explanation.

4. Take notes. In the privacy of your home you will want to review in your mind the things you have been told. You will not remember details if you do not take notes. Though it seemed perfectly clear when the doctor went over the cause of the problem, or why he is recommending a particular approach to treatment, when you try to explain it to your husband or wife it may not seem nearly as reasonable. Taking notes is invaluable in this situation, and you may find that you need another session to clarify points you and the doctor may have missed.

5. Ask specific questions. When you are trying to establish the impact of the illness or injury on your life-style, you must ask questions that will give you answers relevant to your life-style. Otherwise, the information you get may be much too general, and you will feel angry and frustrated. For example, if you want to know if you can continue mountain climbing despite your recent diagnosis of emphysema, you should ask, "Can I continue to climb mountains at 12,000 feet elevation?" not, "Can I continue my usual exercise?" which would likely give you a misleading answer.

6. Recognize and conquer your fear of the future and of the unknown. We all have this tendency. It may be convenient and less painful at the moment not to think about the future, but it is necessary to know the course of an illness in order to plan for what is likely to occur, especially if the disease is progressive. Similarly, one can ignore a sign or symptom (a lump, a sore, a pain, weight loss) for a while, but if it persists more than a couple of weeks it is not likely to go away by itself. Often the truth is less serious than our secret dreads and fantasies. And since almost all serious problems grow with time, it is much easier to treat them when they are still small problems.

7. Do not press for answers that do not exist. The doctor can only give you general statements about many things you probably want to know about your illness or injury. Statistics about the course of the illness, the number of people who die from the illness, the possibility of side effects from medication, etc., are just that— statistics. Statistics are derived from large groups of people who have had the same medical problem and cannot predict what will happen in your individual case. The same illness never follows exactly the same course in any two people, so it is impossible to tell an individual person exactly what his future will hold. Be very careful in looking at any statistics. Even if a certain cancer has only a ten percent chance of cure, if you happen to be in the ten percent, the other ninety percent is really irrelevant; of course, the same would be true in the opposite circumstances! By the same token, a five percent chance of serious side effects from an arthritis medication may be worth the risk when weighed against the potential benefit of pain relief and improved life-style made possible by taking the medication. Weigh all such comparisons carefully; statistics can give you a general feeling for your situation but can predict nothing specifically for you.

◆ Mike prepared for his second visit to his doctor and felt fairly relaxed and calm as he thought about the sort of questions he needed to ask to get enough information to deal with his high blood pressure and to learn to keep it under control with appropriate treatment. Yet as he sat in the waiting room, he suddenly felt panicky. Could he really ask the doctor all these questions? He seemed to be a busy doctor, and maybe he just did not have time to spend on someone with a simple case of high blood pressure. Maybe he should just cancel the appointment.

Cancelling the appointment would be a real mistake for Mike. He has questions about his medical problem, no matter how small it may seem, and he is not going to feel comfortable until the questions are answered and his concerns are addressed. However small the problem may seem, if it is not resolved in the patient's mind, it deserves more discussion. It is a real mistake for people to avoid talking to their doctors about medical problems because they feel their illnesses are small compared to those of others. This often happens though, in part because they are uncertain about their relationships with their doctors and what is expected of them or what is allowed in that relationship.

The relationship that one develops with his family doctor is often a very close relationship. The doctor may be privy to more intimate details of the patient's life than even close family members. And, like any relationship, that between a doctor and patient requires nurturing and mutual trust and, most of all, good ongoing communication by both parties. This relationship is critical when there is ongoing illness or complications related to serious injury, because of the inevitable ups and downs of the medical problem and its impact and ramifications on the patient's and the family's life over many years.

Often it is easier for people to maintain and develop a good relationship with a doctor if they have a set of guidelines to follow in establishing that interaction. That way they can know what they can reasonably expect from the doctor and what he can expect from them. The following, we feel, are a set of such guidelines. They list in general terms rights and responsibilities for both doctors and patients.

We will begin with patient rights and responsibilities. A patient has a right to whatever information he wishes about his illness. The doctor is paid by the patient to facilitate a diagnosis and appropriate therapy, but the medical condition is suffered by the patient and he is the one who has to cope with the future consequences. If he does not wish information, he should communicate this to the doctor. However, this is usually not the case, nor the best course of action.

A second right is that of adequate access to the physician. We have already talked about the need to make a follow-up appointment to get more basic information about one's problem, but access beyond that is important too. Most chronic conditions require regular follow-up and reassessment. This may mean weekly, monthly, quarterly, or even annual visits; whatever is appropriate to the situation.

The patient has a right to and should be encouraged to participate in major decisions relevant to his care. This may involve decisions about different approaches to making a diagnosis (e.g., alternative testing procedures), deciding on alternative forms of therapy, or even if the patient wishes to institute therapy at all. Factors about which the doctor may have no knowledge may be of utmost importance in your life-style. A model with asthma may be able to take her medication only at certain times of the day because of her work and could achieve much better control of her illness if her medications were adjusted to fit this constraint.

When an irretrievable breakdown occurs in a relationship with his doctor, the patient has a right/responsibility to change physicians; however, a comfortable relationship with a doctor takes time and work, and changing doctors should only be done when efforts to resolve the conflicts have failed. Most often relationships sour because of a failure of communication or a misunderstanding, and a simple call or a bit of effort on either party's part can resolve the difficulty; the doctor may not even realize the patient is unhappy! Issues which can usually not be resolved include those involving philosophical differences, ethical conflicts, or personality characteristics of the doctor which annoy the patient and are not likely to change.

The patient needs to know the provisions for coverage that the physician has arranged when he is not available, and he needs to meet these other doctors to make sure he can work with them if the need arises; illness unfortunately has a habit of striking on weekends, holidays, and nights!

The patient has a right to confidentiality of his records, except in cases where the doctor is required by law to report illness that may be a threat to others in certain circumstances. Tuberculosis is one such disease which is communicable and therefore may threaten the public health, so cases must be reported to health authorities.

Any charges for which you will be responsible should be explained to you before you see the doctor. If you are unable to afford the charges, you then have the opportunity to see someone else or to negotiate a lesser charge or payment schedule.

Finally, a person is entitled to be seen within a reasonable time of the scheduled appointment. It is important to remember that sometimes patients preceding you in the schedule may have presented unforeseen problems to the doctor. That kind of situation might require the doctor's immediate attention, with the result being some delay in his schedule. This sort of situation cannot be helped. Some doctors, however, are habitually late; you must decide in your own circumstance what you will or will not tolerate. This is a characteristic unlikely to change, and if you find it sufficiently annoying, you may wish to choose a different doctor.

The patient's rights in his relationship with his physician are attended by an accompanying set of responsibilities.

To make a correct diagnosis and initiate appropriate therapy, the patient must disclose to the doctor all facts about his symptoms and personal life that might be relevant to his health. If the doctor misses a bump or fails to ask about a symptom, this may have been an oversight, and the patient should volunteer the information. It may be irrelevant, but it may just as well be important and could help the doctor to make the diagnosis more quickly, or with fewer tests, or even to make the correct diagnosis.

The patient has a responsibility to plan his visit. It is important for you to think about your symptoms before your appointment. How long has the lump been there? Is it getting larger? Does it itch? Does it hurt? Are there other related symptoms? And so on. The more accurate and precise a description you can give, the easier and faster it will be for the doctor to help you. The history is often ninety percent of the diagnosis!

When a diagnosis has been reached, it is not only your right, but also your responsibility, to understand in detail what is wrong with you and what treatment is available and planned for you. So if you do not understand or explanations are not clear, you should ask for a simpler, more detailed, or clearer description, whichever seems to be appropriate. Ask questions! It is important for both you and the doctor to know how you perceive your condition so that your care can be tailored to your needs.

Once a plan is set up to reach a diagnosis, or a diagnosis is made and a plan for ongoing care is outlined, it is important for the patient to adhere as closely as possible to the plan and report quickly any new symptoms or complications from medication or tests. If such a plan has been worked out with the participation of the patient, instructions should be relatively easy to follow; however, if there is some reason that the plan cannot be carried out or needs modification, a new approach should be worked out by the patient and doctor together.

Some seemingly minor responsibilities really amount to common courtesy, but are the sort of thing that if neglected can cause smoldering resentment and eventual disruption of an otherwise successful relationship. These responsibilities include keeping scheduled appointments or cancelling at least twenty-four hours in advance, limiting intervisit phone calls to important matters, keeping such calls short, and finally, paying bills promptly or in a way that has been mutually agreed upon in advance.

In his role in the relationship, the physician has certain rights and responsibilities as well. In many ways these complement those of the patient. Probably the most important right and responsibility of the doctor is to act professionally in the best interest of the patient. To do this, he/she needs and has the right to full disclosure of information by the patient regarding the patient's health, adequate time to conduct necessary tests or other evaluations to reach a most likely diagnosis, and prompt notification of any worsening of symptoms or other factors affecting the overall health of the patient.

The doctor has the right and moral responsibility to withdraw from the care of a patient who asks him to do something which he/she feels is unethical or if a personality conflict or emotional involvement exists. In such a circumstance, if the patient is in need of immediate care, he/she should help to make arrangements for ongoing care by another physician. An example of such a situation might be the philosophy of care of a dying cancer patient. The family or patient might request withdrawal of active treatment at some point; the doctor might be philosophically opposed to withdrawing treatment and may suggest that the patient change to a physician who feels more comfortable following his wishes.

Probably the physician's right that is most often violated by patients, is the right to privacy and free time. When not in his/her office or on call, the doctor is a private citizen with a private life. This time needs to be respected by patients. The doctor will have made arrangements for someone on-call to cover the practice, and that is the person who should be contacted when the doctor is off duty; that doctor will have access to all your records and will be able to deliver adequate care until your physician is again available.

As with rights, responsibilities of the physician in the doctor-patient relationship often parallel or complement the patient responsibilities.

It is the responsibility of the physician to discuss thoroughly the diagnosis, tests, and treatment plans in a nontechnical way that the average lay person can understand. He/she should encourage questions from the patient. A good way to ensure that the patient has an adequate understanding and perception is to have him repeat back what he understands to be the problem, the proposed treatment, possible complications, prognosis, and so on. This is an especially useful technique for patients who have difficulty formulating appropriate questions, or who are very shy.

Often, alternative approaches to reaching a diagnosis or instituting therapy are possible. In such circumstances, the physician should present reasonable alternatives to the patient. The doctor should also recommend what he/she feels is the best approach to take; this, however, may not be the ultimate path chosen, as lifestyle or other concerns peculiar to that particular patient may become apparent and a mutually acceptable compromise will be necessary.

The doctor is responsible for informing his patients of the provisions for non-office hour coverage, and at some point arranging for patients who so wish, to meet the doctors covering the off time. A doctor must keep good patient records and assist patients in obtaining ancillary services—such as physiotherapy—when such treatment is warranted. He/she is also responsible for informing patients of services that will not be covered by insurance, before the services are rendered, so that any misunderstandings can be averted.

Probably the most difficult, but one of the most important of the physician's responsibilities, is to be able to recognize when he is in over his head. There is no physician who at some time is not unsure of a diagnosis, the reading of an x ray, or what way to proceed next with a patient who is not responding to therapy. It is necessary for the physician to recognize when help is needed and to, at that point, call in a specialist for consultation, or to request a second opinion, or simply to discuss the case with a colleague. This does not mean that the family doctor gives up the patient's care to someone else; quite the contrary, the specialist or doctor offering the second opinion should make recommendations to the referring family doctor and assist the family doctor in carrying out appropriate care.

The above guidelines probably do not cover all aspects of your relationship with your doctor, but they should give you a general framework in which to function and feel comfortable without worrying about taking too much time or overstepping your bounds. As each individual doctor-patient relationship grows, factors unique to that interaction will define the ultimate boundaries and rules.

◆ Uncertainty about what he could ask was not the only problem Mike had in preparing for his second visit to his doctor. Indeed, he knew so little about high blood pressure and illness in general that he had difficulty deciding exactly what kind of things he needed to ask about. He was also scared that he might forget something important and suffer complications because of his ignorance.

Many people feel at a complete loss as to what questions to ask the doctor, because few of us spend time thinking about being or becoming ill. Even those of us who are highly educated, panic when faced with a mountain of medical information that may be as hard to decipher as theoretical physics! Even more frightening than the unintelligible abyss of multisyllable words is describing in revealing detail something that is *wrong* with that which is most intimate to us, our bodies! It's a very vulnerable and insecure feeling.

It need not be so! There are a few basic questions, all of which can be answered in plain English (or whatever your language) that anyone can understand. These are questions that one should ask regardless of what the illness or injury is, and the answers when taken together should give a good overview and basic understanding of the medical problem. When getting information about any medical condition, the general areas one needs to cover are (1) cause (etiology) of the process, (2) course(s) that the disease process or injury might take, and (3) approaches to therapy. Here again, it is best to be organized when asking questions and to cover each of the three areas fully before moving to the next. Moving from cause to treatment and back to cause, for example, can be very confusing and the information will be much harder to understand and remember.

The following section contains a list of important questions you need to cover for a full understanding of your medical problem. The first set of questions deals with etiology.

◆ **What is the cause of my illness?** This may be an easy or difficult question. You may have had a stroke because of your uncontrolled high blood pressure and the cause is easily explained; or you may have an uncommon disease of unknown cause (called idiopathic). In this latter case, you may never know exactly what the cause is. It is much more difficult to visualize and cope with disease of uncertain or unknown cause. Unfortunately, medical science still has many unsolved mysteries, and sometimes the data available even on common diseases is less than satisfying. It is useful to ask for illustrations or drawings of your injury or mechanism of disease, or the area of an organ(s) involved in such diseases as cancer. For many of us, a picture really is worth a thousand words! If the disease is an infection or if it is inherited (genetic), it is important to ask further questions. In the case of infections, you need to ask: "Can this illness be passed to others?" and "What precautions should be taken to prevent the spread of the illness to others?"

In the case of hereditary problems, the type of genetic passage is important so that counseling of family members who might have the disease or who might pass the disease to children can be undertaken.

More pervasive and less clear are those diseases that do not seem to have clear genetic transmission, yet seem to occur in some families more than in others. Some of these illnesses include asthma, high blood pressure, breast cancer, autoimmune diseases, and diabetes mellitus. Thus even when a disease is not clearly an inherited disease, it is useful to ask: "Is there an increased chance that other members of my family will develop this disease since I have it?"

The next area to ask about is that of the course of the medical problem. Information about the course of an illness is critical not only to the person suffering the illness, but also to the family who will inevitably be affected by the process. It is necessary to ask specific questions in order to get as specific an answer as possible. Decisions that may affect one's entire future may be made based on what is thought to be the likely course of the disease. The lives of an entire family are often thrown into disarray when an illness strikes, and it is crucial to the survival of that family to be able to restructure the future to accommodate the illness. To do that, they must have some idea of what is likely to be the course of the disease.

This is an area where doctors do not like to commit themselves because, certainly, none of us can predict the future for any single other person. The usual course of diseases is derived from following large numbers of persons with that illness over time, and then calculating statistics of complications, survival, good response to treatment, poor response to treatment, and so on. Any single person may have quite a different course—he might do much better or much worse—than the averages described by statistics.

Another reason that doctors are reluctant to predict what will happen in a particular person's situation, especially if the patient is likely to have a rapid and progressive course, is that they do not like to take hope away from the ill person, leaving him despondent and depressed. Nevertheless, for the person's future planning for himself and his family, it is necessary to understand the full spectrum of any disease. This may allow early job retraining, revision of retirement plans, or in the worst scenarios, appropriate planning for the family after the ill person's death.

Some of the important specific questions you should ask to help define for you the likely course of your illness or injury are:

◆ **Is this disease progressive?** In what way? Will I lose the function of the organs involved, and will other organs become involved? Will this disease shorten my life?

◆ **Can I become disabled or disfigured by this problem or by the treatment?**

◆ **Is there any complication I might develop from the disease or treatment that would make me unable to work as a _____?**

◆ **How will I know if a serious complication is developing?**

◆ **Are there complications of the disease that might interfere with my life-style?** In asking this question, obviously the doctor must know enough about you to give a meaningful answer. If he/she does not, you must be more specific about the information you want. If you fly small planes as a hobby and you want to know the potential effect on your flying ability, you must ask specifically about flying. Any specific sports, social activities, travel plans, or other life events should be individually addressed.

The third area that is important to explore with your doctor is that of treatment. As already mentioned, in most cases the therapy of adult disease is not aimed at cure because most adult illnesses are not curable. However, in most instances symptoms are treatable, and in a group of illnesses, the course of the illness can be slowed or stopped by appropriate medication or care. Unfortunately, almost all medications have side effects; but most of these are usually just nuisances. That is, they are unpleasant but not dangerous. Others, though, might be toxic or dangerous to other organs, and it is important to understand exactly what these potential toxicities are before taking any medication. At times, alternative therapies may be available, e.g., surgery, physiotherapy, other drugs. It is necessary to learn about the alternative approaches to therapy before the decisions are made in order to tailor your treatment appropriately. Thus, you should not begin a prescribed course of treatment blindly until you have had answered:

◆ **Are there any alternative treatments for my condition, and what are the reasons for recommending my specific therapy?**

More information regarding side effects of medications and medication interactions are covered in Chapter 2 of this section.

Chronic and particularly progressive illness often demands repeated visits to one or more doctors, and these visits can be quite frequent. Thus it is very important in such a situation, that you have a doctor in whom you have confidence. The need for continuous medical care fosters an even closer relationship with the doctor than that which normally develops when a family doctor is being consulted for a variety of problems.

That need for ongoing care for a debilitating or potentially debilitating problem can cause a great deal of frustration for the patient, if the doctor does not respond to an individual's needs in an expected way, or as rapidly or completely as the person feels is necessary. Someone who is suffering increasing symptoms or debility is very vulnerable. He wishes the illness to go away and leave him whole again, but often this cannot happen and, unfortunately, the doctor cannot alter that. The patient may erroneously interpret the doctor's inability to get rid of the illness, or the doctor's trying of several different approaches at therapy in an attempt to find a successful one for the patient, as his not knowing what he is doing or as withholding information about the illness. Often in chronic illness, the course for each person is different, and the doctor cannot give specific answers or concrete statements about what the effect of a specific therapy will be; answers simply do not exist, and most often cures do not exist either. However, some doctors are better at communicating with their chronically ill patients than are others. They take the time at each visit to answer questions and chat. It is a common complaint, however, for patients with chronic illness to feel that their doctor is not communicating or is not answering questions specifically enough. They don't feel a personal connection. Sometimes this is true. Many doctors want to have the answers and the cures, and fall silent when they can't be hopeful or positive. Judge for yourself. It is important to feel that your doctor is taking the time to communicate with you. It is important to feel completely safe and confident in him or her.

These frustrations, understandably, may be expressed in feelings of anger directed toward the doctor because he/she is perceived as the one who cannot cure the illness. It is really anger at the illness itself, but since the illness has no physical form, it becomes much easier to organize one's feelings toward a person who is associated with the illness. Sometimes these feelings reach such a point that the relationship with the doctor is destroyed; and if this happens, even if the underlying anger is recognized, it may be necessary to change doctors.

In other long-term doctor-patient relationships, a patient can become very attached to a single doctor who "knows my story," and may feel very insecure in anyone else's care. While this is understandable, it is important to realize that no one can be available twenty-four hours a day, seven days a week, and it is important to get to know the other doctors who will be covering your doctor's practice when he/she is away.

Nevertheless, the strong attachments that develop can result in some common but dysfunctional situations. It is not unusual when you know your doctor is going on vacation, for example, to develop worsening symptoms or new symptoms, in the several days around that time. This can happen as well when a doctor moves away or dies. Sometimes it happens as often as every Friday when a patient realizes his/her doctor may not be available for two days! Often these symptoms are related to anxiety and fears that the doctor who is trusted will not be there if you get sick. While that may be true, someone who can care for you will be. Recognizing this and reassuring yourself of it, or clarifying this with the doctor who will care for you, usually relieves these concerns.

Some patients always feel worse when they are at home than when they are at the doctor's office or in the hospital, even though the treatment in the hospital may be no more than can be carried out at home. Again, these feelings often arise because of anxiety or fear that somehow, if one is in the hospital, he cannot get worse or die. This, of course, is not rational, but it can be a very powerful feeling. If you find yourself wanting not to go home from the hospital, or feeling much more comfortable in the hospital, these fears or anxieties are likely what is underlying your feelings. Sometimes it is a close family member, rather than the ill person, who is harboring these feelings. He/she may feel very uncomfortable and responsible with the person at home.

The first step in dealing with this situation is to recognize that this is what is happening. The next step is getting a clear idea from the doctor about what to expect in terms of worsening symptoms and what sort of symptoms should prompt you to call him/her. Find out how long a new symptom, e.g., pain or fever, should be allowed to persist before medical care is sought. Find out what to expect from medications in terms of treating symptoms and how to recognize the signs of serious side effects. And finally, make sure you understand how to get ahold of the doctor or his/her colleagues at any time, day or night. In the case of a doctor's moving away, make sure you know who will be taking over the practice well in advance of the move, and meet the person so you know if you can work with him/her, or if not, have plenty of time to find someone new.

If this sort of preparation does not reduce your fears and anxieties to a manageable level, a professional counselor may be helpful. One often successful approach is to use relaxation techniques that can be learned from a counselor, or from a number of audiocassette tapes that are available. (See Chapter 9, Managing Personality Changes, for more about relaxation training.)

◆ All of us are shocked when we get a diagnosis of any kind of illness. Our natural self-protective mechanism is to shut out potentially harmful news, so we often remember little of what the doctor tells us. It is important to make follow-up appointments to find out more about the illness.

◆ You will gain more from doctor's visits if you think about your symptoms ahead of time, organize your thoughts, and go prepared.

◆ The relationship between doctor and patient is complex and very important. Patients may feel intimidated because they do not know how to act in such a relationship. It is necessary to establish ground rules and stick to them if the relationship is to last and grow.

◆ It is important to ask certain questions about any illness, in order to understand the impact that illness is likely to have on your life. These can be written down and taken with you on your visits so you will get all the necessary information.

◆ It is important to be able to communicate freely with your doctor and to feel that he/she is taking the time to speak with you and answer your questions.

◆ Chronic illnesses carry with them special considerations with respect to the doctor-patient relationship. Vulnerability, fear, and anxiety can create uncomfortable situations for people suffering these illnesses. Recognizing the fears often helps in coping with them, though professional counseling may be necessary.

CHAPTER 2

Adjusting to Medication
and Other Therapy

Thousands of medications are available and heavily advertised by a very large pharmaceutical industry. Some of these drugs are literally life-saving, others effective in varying degrees in different people, and still others hardly useful at all. Among the most confusing and difficult issues in coping with chronic illness is achieving the optimum results from appropriate medication. To find the best drugs with the least obnoxious side effects from among the variety that are usually available for any given ailment, is a real challenge for you and your doctor. Sometimes the period necessary to arrive at optimal therapy can be quite prolonged and can demand an undue amount of your time. Centering one's life around the drugs, and hence around the illness, can easily occur in this setting, and you must be careful to keep some perspective on the situation. Issues of this type will be discussed in succeeding chapters in Section 2.

In this chapter we will look at a number of aspects of drug therapy and other treatments, and discuss how to balance benefits versus risks and how to make informed decisions.

◆ Mike (the gentleman from Chapter 1 who recently discovered he had high blood pressure) had several successive measurements of his blood pressure, and all were felt to be high enough to require drug therapy. His doctor recommended treatment and gave Mike a prescription with instructions about taking the drug. Mike, however, felt well and took the drug only occasionally. Three months later, he returned for follow-up and was found to have an even higher blood pressure than previously.

Two serious errors in the prescribing and taking of medication have occurred here. The first is that the doctor failed to explain fully to Mike the need to take the medication on a regular basis because of the nature of his illness, and he failed to explain fully the nature of the illness, i.e., that it will not go away by itself. The second error was that Mike did not follow the instructions given with the medication, so it did not work. This is called noncompliance, and it usually occurs because the patient does not understand the reason for his medication, the nature of his illness, or does not appreciate the serious complications that can occur if the drug is not used. Sometimes a patient also fails to take medication because of side effects that he finds intolerable. Anytime you begin a medication, you must understand why you are being asked to take it. If you feel you have not had an adequate explanation, you must ask the doctor:

◆ **Why are you prescribing this medication and how will it work in my illness? Are there alternative approaches to therapy?**

(Other issues, like side effects and drug interactions, will be covered later on in this chapter.)

Medications are given for a variety of reasons. When antibiotics cure an infection or pain medications give relief, it is easy to measure the positive effects; however, many medications may have much less readily measurable impact. Antihypertensive (high blood pressure) medication, such as that given Mike, are given for prophylaxis to prevent complications from the underlying disease. In diseases like this, where medication is given to try to prevent future complications, it is very important for the person to understand the need for compliance with medication or he/she will not take it regularly. Once a serious, nonreversible complication occurs—in high blood pressure, it might be a stroke—it is too late.

◆ After discussing the role of his drug, Mike had a much better understanding of his need to take it, and he did—for awhile. However, his job became quite busy, and he often just forgot to take the middle-of-the-day pill. (His pills were to be taken three times a day.) At another visit to have his blood pressure checked, his pressure was high. Mike, somewhat sheepishly, explained to the doctor how hard it was for him to get in three pills a day.

There is no reason to feel sheepish about a situation like this. Life-style is a very important consideration in prescribing not only the best kind of medication, but also one that has a dosing schedule the patient will likely be able to follow. Often it takes several visits and may take several medication trials before either a suitable drug or suitable dosing schedule is found. Luckily, for many illnesses, several alternative drugs or therapies are available that are reasonably good, and the best option for a particular patient can be chosen. That is why when several persons all with the same illness compare their treatments, they are likely to find many differences, though all treatments are probably equally good.

Sometimes in initial discussions with the doctor, a patient will recognize that he/she is likely to have difficulty in taking a suggested drug. It is, of course, important to voice concerns if that happens, so that an unnecessary or traumatic trial with the drug is not undertaken. Another important thing to recognize is that drugs often lessen symptoms but do not prevent or alleviate them completely. If the patient has been expecting one hundred percent relief but gets only eighty percent, he/she may be disenchanted and intolerant of minor side effects. To avoid an unfortunate situation where the patient is disillusioned because of unrealistic expectations, it is useful to ask before starting the treatment: "What amount of relief of my symptoms or slowing of the progression of my illness can I expect?" or "Will this drug likely make me symptom free?"

◆ Mike's doctor was able to switch him to a different type of medication which required only twice-a-day dosing. This was much more acceptable to Mike's life-style. His problems were not over though. Within a few weeks of the time he started on the new medication, he began to have problems achieving an erection. Could this be related to his high blood pressure, the stress at work, or the medication? He hated to go back again to the doctor, so he decided to just drop the drug down to one pill a day, and the problem mostly resolved. But, as you might expect, on his next blood pressure check, the blood pressure was up again! By this time, the doctor had learned to carefully check Mike's drug-taking patterns, and this revealed not only the unacceptable side effect, but also Mike's ill-advised solution.

This situation, which could have had very unfortunate consequences, again resulted because of inadequate information and poor communication between Mike and his doctor. The doctor should always explain potential side effects of medication. If he/she does not, before you leave the office with a new prescription, you must ask: "Does this medication have any side effects that I need to watch for and are any of them potentially dangerous?"

Side effects may be a nuisance, and one may need to live with them if the benefit of the drug outweighs the discomfort, e.g., the shakiness often seen in patients who take cyclosporine for organ transplant immune suppression. Or the side effects may be annoying but are temporary and will wear off in a few days or weeks, and therefore can be tolerated. For Mike, the side effect he experienced was not tolerable and therefore unacceptable, unless no other possible effective alternative therapy could be found. Sometimes side effects can be lessened by a change in the way a drug is taken, e.g., taking a nausea-producing drug with food might relieve nausea. However, such changes are not always appropriate and may make the drug ineffective, as did Mike's self-adjustment of his medication. If a side effect that is annoying occurs, it is always important to inform the doctor so that a solution can be worked out that will not lessen the effect of the drug.

A number of tricks can be used to reduce unpleasant side effects: The common side effect of nausea sometimes can be lessened by taking the medication shortly before bedtime. Bad-tasting drugs can be mixed with pleasant-flavored food or drink but, again, check with the doctor to make sure the food will not inactivate the medicine. Washing one's mouth out with water or a mouthwash after each use, can prevent yeast infections caused by inhaled steroids that are widely used in a variety of lung diseases. Sometimes using enteric-coated (designed to dissolve outside the stomach) or long-acting preparations will reduce stomach discomfort. Changing dosages can occasionally still be effective but relieve such side effects as dizziness, stomach cramps, shakiness, etc. If a side effect occurs that you have not been warned about or that you have been told to recognize as potentially dangerous, you must always inform the doctor promptly, and the two of you can work out a new regimen or alternative therapy. Remember that if the various possibilities for side effects are discussed at the time the drug is prescribed, much grief, ill-feeling, and many urgent phone calls can be prevented!

Toxic or potentially dangerous effects, as distinguished from side effects, refer to the potential of a drug to cause damage to any organ and thereby threaten your overall health. These need to be carefully outlined and explained to you because a number of drugs have a small risk of causing life-threatening complications. Given the risk of toxicity, you must carefully balance this against the likelihood of benefit from the drug and make a decision whether you wish to take the risk of the toxicity. For example, certain nonsteroidal pain relievers can cause severe kidney damage or bleeding from the gut; yet they have a high rate of pain relief for sufferers of arthritis. If you have painful arthritis and live in constant discomfort, it may be worth it for you to take the risk of the medication so that you can live a more pleasant life. On the other hand, a less than one percent risk of death from anesthesia may be enough of a risk to induce you not to have a hernia repair!

If you are taking a drug with potentially harmful effects, you need to ask what sort of symptoms or signs will herald the onset of such an effect and how often you will need routine laboratory monitoring, e.g., blood and urine studies. These studies can often pick up such toxicities early before you might be aware of any signs or symptoms. If caught early enough, many toxic effects can be reversed by stopping a drug or reducing the dosage. Be sure and ask the doctor specifically: "Should I have routine monitoring of my blood or urine?" "How often?"

Allergies to drugs deserve a separate mention. This generally might be considered a toxic effect unique to a specific individual who is sensitized to the components of that drug. It is critical that you tell the doctor about any drug allergies you have experienced in the past, before you begin taking a new medication. Drug allergies can be life-threatening, and sometimes other drugs that are chemically related but have completely different names, can cause the same reaction. Therefore, if the doctor does not know about your drug allergies, you could be prescribed a drug to which you might have a serious allergic reaction, even though you may have never before taken the drug!

◆ Mike finally felt he had things straightened out. He got into a routine, and he never missed his twice-a-day blood pressure pills. His check-ups began to show that his pressure was under good control. He was able to reduce the follow-ups to every three or four months. In fact he was doing so well that, after a couple of years, he decided he was cured and could stop his medication. One day he awoke with a terrible headache and had to go to the emergency room. His blood pressure was dangerously high, and he had to be admitted to the hospital.

It is dangerous to guess at how long a medication or any other therapy needs to be continued. A few are short term, like antibiotics, but many must be continued indefinitely or even for life. Blood pressure medication is usually a lifelong treatment. You should never stop a medication suddenly without first finding out from the doctor if there are complications in doing this. Some blood pressure medications, for example, when stopped suddenly may actually result in a rebound high pressure; other medications taken for long periods of time, like corticosteroids, when stopped suddenly may result in a life-threatening situation.

You should always ask the doctor if there are any special instructions for taking a particular medication. Not stopping the medication suddenly would be one type of special instruction. Other examples of this would be a warning that a drug might cause drowsiness, that the drug should be taken before or after meals, or that a drug should not be taken with certain other drugs. Some drugs sensitize you to the sun and you can get a severe sunburn if you do not use a good sunscreen; some drugs cause a severe reaction when alcohol is used while they are being taken.

Of particular concern are interactions between drugs. Drugs used in the same person to treat different illnesses may interact with each other or may influence the body's removal system so that it works slower or faster. This in turn may result in the presence of excessive or inadequate amounts of the drug being present in your body. To prevent this from happening, the doctor must know about any medications you are already taking so that when he/she prescribes new drugs, ones that might result in such interactions will be avoided. Even so, it is always worth asking: "Is there any possible reaction that can occur between this new drug and the _____ I am already taking?"

A thorough history of all previous illness is also important information for the doctor before he/she recommends new therapies for you. Occasionally, a previous illness that may now be quiescent is exacerbated or reactivated by the use of a new medication. For example, an asthmatic whose lung disease has been inactive can have the recurrence of wheezing or coughing when certain heart or high blood-pressure drugs are started. Other drugs that would not cause this recurrence of symptoms would be available in most cases.

◆ With the scare he received, Mike became religious about taking his pills. If he missed one in the morning, he'd leave work and go home to take it; he bought a blood-pressure cuff and measured his blood pressure twice a day. If it was a little high, he'd take an extra pill.

Thankfully, Mike has learned the benefit of being compliant with his drug regimen. A word of caution, however, is in order. In the face of a near catastrophic event, death of a close relative, or other crisis, one can become fixated on medical problems and obsessed with medication or other factors that might influence health, like diet or environmental issues. This makes the illness or medications, or whatever is fixated upon, the center of one's life. An excessive concern with one's health can be very restricting and disruptive to both the victim and the family, and their social interactions. One must be careful to try to keep a reasonable perspective.

Other Treatments

Certain medical problems have treatment options other than medication. These might include diet restrictions, environmental changes, hydrotherapy, physiotherapy, exercise programs, occupational therapy, or surgery.

In each case, whenever a potential treatment is presented to you, it is important for you to weigh the potential for benefit against the potential risk of taking that action. To find this out you have to ask the appropriate questions. Because of the above-mentioned treatment options, the only one which regularly poses potential serious risk to patients is surgery. Let us spend a few moments on the specific questions that need to be addressed before you make a decision regarding surgery:

◆ How is this surgery expected to help me? Can you draw me a picture of what you are going to do?
◆ What are the chances it will work?
◆ What are my risks of serious complication or death from the surgery? Do I have an increased risk because of my medical condition?
◆ Am I at increased risk of death or complications from anesthesia?
◆ How much time should it take me to recover from this surgery?
◆ What alternatives are there to the surgery and what will likely happen if I do not have it?

If the procedure suggested carries a high risk or alternative treatment options are available, it may be desirable to obtain a second or specialist opinion to help you make a decision. More information about obtaining this kind of help is included in Chapter 3.

Optimal control of illness or injury symptoms and disabilities allows the patient and the family to better tackle the overwhelming psychological aspects of medical problems. But to do this, one must first thoroughly understand the illness and the aims of therapy.

◆ Not taken according to directions, medications can at the best be ineffective, and at the worst deadly. It is important both for the doctor to explain carefully the role of the medication, and for the patient to take it exactly as directed.

◆ Life-style should be taken into account as much as possible when medication is prescribed to enable the patient to adhere to medication instructions. To make sure this is done, the doctor and patient should thoroughly discuss the patient's situation before a drug is prescribed.

◆ Potential side effects of medication should be thoroughly discussed and understood before taking any medication. Dangerous side effects should be distinguished from less significant side effects. Instructions for what to do in case of the occurrence of side effects should be given.

◆ It is important to let the doctor know if you are taking any medication that he/she has not prescribed, because some drugs interact with each other or alcohol and are not compatible. It is also necessary to make the doctor aware of any previous drug allergies; sometimes ingredients are contained in drugs you are being prescribed that are similar to one to which you are allergic and might cause an allergy.

◆ Do not stop taking medication or change the dose without consulting the doctor first.

CHAPTER 3

Testing, Consulting, and Second Opinions: When and Why?

For those of us who are lucky, our medical problems will improve spontaneously or respond quickly to treatment and remain quiescent or stable for many years. However, many of us will not be so fortunate, and as the years pass, we will have increasing interaction with the medical system. Because many illnesses progress or complications develop or our aging bodies develop new diseases, the complexity of the necessary medical care we require is ever increasing. This can be frightening and confusing.

Undoubtedly if you have chronic illness, you will at some time be confronted with requests by your doctor to undergo one or a number of tests or procedures in attempts to clarify the extent of illness, or to monitor the effect of therapy. The technology of medicine has become so advanced that by using various testing procedures, it is often possible to make quite precise measurements or almost "see" the internal organs of the body affected by disease. Another issue that might arise as your illness becomes worse or if any type of difficulties appears, is whether or not other doctors should be called upon. This can involve specialist consultation or the obtaining of second opinions. This chapter will help you to decide when and if you should agree to or initiate requests for this type of care.

Before you agree to anything, you need information. You should understand basically why a test or consultation has been requested and exactly what the item that has been requested would involve. To explore some of these issues, let us follow Mike (Chapters 1 and 2) a little further along in his life.

◆ Mike had learned to live with his high blood pressure which he had for about ten years. Now at age 52, Mike apparently had another problem that Dr. Mills said could be a complication of his high blood pressure. The results of a physical examination and a chest x ray showed that he had a large heart, and Dr. Mills said he needed more tests. Mike was really scared now; a guy at work had just dropped dead of a heart attack. Was he going to be next?

The first thing to do when you hear, "We need some tests . . ." is not panic. Get information.

You first need to understand some general concepts about tests. In every test or procedure, you must in some way be able to balance the potential benefit of that test against the potential risk. Generally, tests can be classified as either noninvasive or invasive. Noninvasive studies generally do not involve actually entering or "invading" the body, and so are usually less risky. Invasive studies, on the other hand, are studies that are more complex and require entering a body space. Therefore, the risk is usually greater and in some cases may even include risk of death from an unexpected complication.

Noninvasive studies would include, for example, electrocardiograms (ECG), routine x-ray studies, or ultrasound studies where a microphone placed on the body surface is used to reflect sound waves off internal structures, which in turn provide images of the internal structures.

Invasive studies might include tests in which instruments equipped with fiber-optics are passed via the esophagus or airways to visualize the interior of these structures. Other examples of invasive studies are catheterizations of (or the placing of hollow tubes into) blood vessels to assess coronary artery and other vessel disease, and the taking of small pieces of tissue (biopsies) from organs, so that the tissues can be examined under a microscope for any changes indicating disease. Bleeding or subsequent infection can be serious risks of such studies.

Since the risk of invasive studies can be significant, it is important that in this type of study you give written informed consent. Prior to any procedure which poses significant risk in terms of either complications or mortality, the doctor is obligated to explain the procedure in terms you can understand, and to list for you all of the possible complications of the test. If you do not understand the procedure or the risks, or you are not willing to take the risks, you should not sign the informed consent form. The consent should be signed before you are given any premedication drugs that might cause you to be groggy and not fully aware of what you are doing.

Despite these necessary precautions and protection of your rights, do not lose sight of the fact that your doctor will not be recommending to you a potentially risky procedure unless he/she really feels it is going to reveal something important about your condition and will aid in giving you the optimal care. Risks of a procedure vary widely—from far less than one percent to greater than fifty percent. No one can predict when a complication will occur. Nevertheless, you must always try to balance the potential benefit of the test against the risks that might sound ominous, but might occur with very low frequency. Usually if the information needed might be gotten by less invasive means, the doctor will try these first.

The prospect of undergoing almost any test is intimidating. You often have to take off all or part of your clothes, and this makes you feel very vulnerable because the person testing you is not going to be half-naked! What's worse, something bad might be discovered in the test; something that is wrong with you and that might not be able to be fixed! That's doubly scary.

It's difficult to get rid of all these uncomfortable feelings because, no matter how you package it, a test is usually unpleasant. However, you can reduce your anxiety to a minimum if you can find out as much information as possible before the test. Some practical matters should be sorted out first. Tests are expensive and can be time consuming. Find out how much the tests will cost and if they will be covered by your health insurance. Find out if you will need to be hospitalized and, if so, you will probably have to make arrangements to be off work for a few days or to have child care or whatever your special circumstances require. The following is a list of useful questions that will help to ease your mind, and the answers should ensure that you understand what you are getting into with your proposed test(s):

◆ How will this test aid in the diagnosis or therapy of my condition?

◆ Will the results give an answer or might I have to have further studies done? If so, when would they need to be done?

◆ Do I have any particular risks because of my medical condition, or for any other reasons?

◆ Could other, less uncomfortable or less risky ways be used to get the same information?

In addition to these general questions, you should get more specific information about the test you are about to undergo. Knowing in advance the details of the procedure will greatly relieve your greatest fear, that of the unknown. You will find that with this type of information in advance, most tests are not nearly as bad as you imagined them. Thus, to avoid unpleasant surprises during or after the test, and to make sure that you do not inadvertently do something that will interfere with the test results, you will need to find out the following:

◆ Ask the doctor to explain exactly what will happen during the test in a step-by-step fashion.
◆ Ask if premedication will be given, and what you should expect to feel like after it is given.
◆ Ask if any type of anesthesia will be used, and if complications from it could occur.
◆ Find out the approximate length of the test.
◆ Find out the incidence of risk of the test and an estimate of your particular risk.
◆ Ask about special instructions that must be followed in preparing for the test, or after the test is completed.
◆ Ask whether you should expect to feel any unusual sensations or pain during or after the test.
◆ Ask how to recognize complications of the test or premedication, and what you should do if they happen.

◆ Make arrangements for follow-up to get results of the test and to plan for future care.

With this information you will be better able to participate in your ongoing care, and you must do this to maintain some control over your life situation. The better you understand your overall health problems, the better you'll be able to cope with whatever comes along.

◆ One of the tests that Mike did was called an exercise stress test. To do the test, electrocardiogram leads were taped to Mike's chest and his heartbeat was watched on a monitor while Mike exercised on a treadmill. Mike found that as he did more and more exercise, a tight feeling came across his chest and soon the doctor stopped the test. Later he told Mike that there were some changes on his ECG during the exercise, and he would like to send him to a cardiologist to get a better idea about how to handle this new problem and to decide if any further tests should be done. Now what would Mike do? He had come to feel very comfortable with Dr. Mills, who knew him better than anyone. He really did not want a different doctor, but at the same time he wanted to have the best care available. He felt a good deal of anxiety about what this new problem would mean to his future, and about what else a specialist might find.

Many people with chronic illness will at some time during the disease be facing just the situation that Mike is. Specialist consultation or a second opinion may be advisable in a number of circumstances, yet this is also often anxiety producing because it often signals a worsening of the disease or some problem with therapy. It is also anxiety producing because it means we will have to establish some sort of relationship with another doctor, and we are worried about whether we will like him/her, how this new doctor will approach our problems, etc. It is natural also to feel some ambivalence about engaging in this new relationship because most of us have developed a good relationship with our family or primary doctor, and we are concerned that that relationship might be harmed if a specialist becomes involved.

A specialist is a doctor who has taken special advanced training in a particular area of medicine or surgery. It is important to recognize that the specialist is really a consultant and will probably see you only once. Occasionally, if you have a particularly severe disease or a particularly difficult problem with your disease, he may follow you at intermittent intervals. However, the main function of the specialist is to assist your primary physician in your care. After seeing you, the specialist will send back recommendations to your family physician and work with him/her. Despite specialist or second opinion input, your primary relationship remains with your family doctor. In most cases, specialist opinions are welcomed. Often the doctor will request the consultation. While second opinions more often are requested by the patient, they too at times are sought by your primary doctor.

The real question in most people's minds is when it is legitimate to bring a specialist in or to get a second opinion. The following list includes circumstances in which specialist consultants are often asked to see a patient, either by the primary doctor or by the patient himself:

◆ If the patient is having rapid progression of the disease or if he/she has failed to respond to the usual therapy of the disease, complication of an injury, etc.
◆ If it is an unusual illness or an unusual manifestation of a common illness that only a specialist could be expected to have much experience in treating.
◆ If a test or procedure is required that must be done by a physician with special training.
◆ If complications or progression of the underlying process develop, which require specialized expertise. (You might, for example, have progression of rheumatoid arthritis to the point that surgery is necessary. Thus an orthopedic surgeon would need to become involved in your care.)

Through the course of a long illness, you might see a number of specialists. It is particularly important in such a circumstance to keep up a good relationship with your primary physician. When too many doctors get involved, you can easily end up being lost in the shuffle. Make sure that your doctor knows when you are seeing a specialist, so that he/she knows when to expect a note from that consultant. In addition, there are some things that you should clarify with your doctor before you see the specialist(s) so that you both know what your expectations are.

If your doctor has initiated the request for consultation, make sure you understand, specifically, the questions he wishes answered by the consultant. While your doctor will send a consultation request to the specialist, sometimes these things get lost, and both you and the consultant can end up wasting a lot of time trying to guess why you are seeing him. It is a good idea to carry a copy of the letter from your doctor to the specialist with you. Other issues that you should discuss with your own doctor before you visit a consultant are:

◆ If changes in approach to therapy (e.g., medication, surgery) are suggested by the specialist, should you comply immediately or only after they have been reviewed by the family doctor?
◆ Does the family doctor wish the consultant to see you only once, or to follow you in subsequent visits?

An important way of assuring that your relationship with your family doctor does not get interrupted is to call and arrange a follow-up visit as soon as you have seen the specialist. Also, make sure that if you are to be hospitalized for surgery, to try new therapy, or whatever, your family doctor is informed so that he/she can participate in that care.

◆ Mike saw the cardiologist who did some more extensive tests, and after reviewing the results, told Mike he thought he should undergo open heart surgery. Mike was very scared by this prospect and thought maybe he would like to try medication or some other approach to therapy first, but if heart surgery was the best option, he would do it. He discussed his fears with Dr. Mills, and they decided to ask for a second opinion.

The issue of seeking a second opinion is slightly different from that of seeking a specialist consultation and may, at times, be a bit more controversial. It is not correct, however, to think of a second opinion as antagonistic toward one's primary physician or specialist. Most doctors fully understand a patient's desire to obtain a second opinion, especially in certain circumstances; in fact, sometimes the doctor will initiate the request. As in the case of specialist consultation, the seeking and obtaining of a second opinion should not interfere with you and your doctor's relationship unless, of course, the issue is one of the competence of your doctor. If you wish to maintain a good ongoing relationship with your doctor, you should tell him/her about your desire to get a second opinion, and warn him/her to expect a letter from the doctor you are seeing for the opinion.

Some situations in which one might wish to seek a second opinion are:

◆ **When the diagnosis is uncertain.** It is often difficult to make a definite diagnosis, especially if the presenting symptoms are not classic. Sometimes another view will either help make the diagnosis or assure you that your own doctor has done everything possible to make a diagnosis. This is also a reason that your own doctor might in some cases ask for specialist consultation.

◆ **If you are not responding to treatment.** Again, occasionally a new view will have a different approach to treatment, or a different doctor may have knowledge of a new drug.

◆ **If you have been advised to undergo particularly risky investigations.** Someone else may suggest alternative studies that are less risky and with which you feel more comfortable, though there is often a trade-off in terms of expected yield.

◆ **If the therapy suggested is risky, experimental, or controversial.** Often multiple approaches to any single problem are available, and some might be better suited to you than others.

◆ **If the diagnosis is that of a fatal illness.** Unfortunately, diagnoses like cancer are usually not equivocal, and are unlikely to change with a second opinion. However, hearing the same thing from two different doctors helps the patient come to grips with the reality of his situation sooner.

Issues centering around the doctor's competence, your confidence in the doctor, or ethical and moral conflicts sometimes also spawn second opinions. The problems here, however, usually signify deep schisms between patient and doctor, and the issue is really one of changing physicians.

You should keep in mind a couple of caveats regarding the question of second opinions. It is important to realize that much of medicine is an art, and that when you get a second opinion that differs from that of your primary doctor or that of another specialist, it does not mean that one is right and the other is wrong. Most often, different opinions simply reflect differences in philosophy or approach to the same problem, although one of the approaches may be more appropriate for your specific situation.

Another thing to be careful about is doctor-hopping. Sometimes when a patient goes for a second opinion, he wants the doctor to say something he wants to hear (like the diagnosis isn't cancer). When he does not hear what he wants, he will find another doctor and another and another, looking for one who will tell him what he wants to hear. Occasionally, if a second opinion differs from that of your original doctor, it is advisable to get a third opinion. But rarely is it helpful to go beyond that; quite the contrary, hopping from one doctor to another can delay therapy and hurt you in the long run.

Tests, consultations, and second opinions need not be frightening. If you have a basic understanding of your medical problems and prepare yourself as described in this chapter, you will feel in control of the situation, and your anxiety will be much reduced.

◆ Before agreeing to undergo tests that are suggested for you, you should understand what information is expected to be gained and how it will help in diagnosing the illness or guiding therapy. Find out if it is a risky test and if there are less risky alternatives.

◆ To allay your fears of the unknown, ask the doctor to explain in detail what will be done during the test so you are not totally unprepared.

◆ Sometimes, specialist consultation will be helpful in your medical care. You may have a rapidly progressive illness, unusual illness, or a complication of your underlying problem, for example, which may be better approached by a person who specializes in the care of persons with diseases similar to yours. It is important to understand the reason for the specialist opinion and the information that your primary doctor expects to gain; your primary relationship should remain with your family doctor.

◆ Certain situations may call for a second opinion. Cases where the diagnosis is uncertain, the disease is not responding to treatment, the diagnosis is life threatening, or the proposed treatment is risky are some common examples. Most doctors are not offended by patients wishing second opinions and may, in fact, ask for one themselves.

CHAPTER 4

Anticipating Medical Crises

One of the pervasive fears of families who live with the daily specter of chronic illness is that a crisis will occur, and they will not know how to handle it. This may be of particular concern to those families where the initial event was sudden—as in the case of a heart attack, stroke, or car accident with spinal-cord injury—yet the event irrevocably changed forever their lives. This experience of total vulnerability and the realization it could happen again can be both frightening and nearly paralyzing.

The possibility of such a crisis is real, though it is not limited to those families who have already suffered such an event. However, it is true that the spectrum of medical crises in families where a debilitating illness already exists is much wider. Complicating acute illnesses, like pneumonia, can in a precipitously short interval place an already ill person in a life-threatening situation.

The best way to cope with this constant possibility is to prepare for it as completely as possible, so that if it should occur, the impact will be lessened. This chapter will outline some important steps in this planning process.

The first step is to talk to your doctor. Ask him/her what the most likely crisis or acute complications might be, which would require immediate attention, and what should be done in each situation (i.e., should he/she be called, should you go by ambulance to the emergency room of the nearest hospital, can you handle it yourself, etc.?). Discuss with your doctor when he/she is available, where he/she sees patients in emergencies, and how long it takes to get there. Find out where the doctor hospitalizes patients and who takes the calls when he/she is not on call; you should meet these people to make sure you can relate to them. The next time you see them, you may be in a very vulnerable or crisis situation.

The next step is to sit down with family members when everything is on an even keel and discuss who will take care of what in an emergency. Talk about what you will need and what to do in the event of a crisis. This might include a way for the ill person to contact help if he/she is alone for long periods of time, a means available on an urgent basis for transportation to medical facilities, baby-sitting help that can be requested on short notice if there are children in the family, household help available on short notice, informing an employer of the possible need to suddenly be away from work, and so on. Single people might need to prearrange for someone to look after pets, certain household chores, or the payment of important bills.

Someone—usually the spouse in families or an adult child in the case of an aging parent, or some other trusted family member— should be designated by the ill person, with the help of his lawyer, to be able to get power of attorney, if this should be necessary in a crisis. This choice should be carefully documented in print and signed. This can be a limited right, but may be used to allow access to funds, carry out necessary business transactions, etc. A prearrangement like this can save families from the annoyance and stress of added financial burdens and urgent business decisions during an already difficult time.

Once all the potential needs of the family in a crisis are identified, a plan of action should be developed. This plan identifies who will do what if a crisis happens. Persons designated to help will thus know in advance of their expected participation, and time will not be lost in indecision and bickering when an event occurs. Also, the family coping with illness will quickly learn who can and cannot be counted on in times of need.

A plan might go something like this. Joe, who has had a stroke and is chairbound at home, develops a blood clot in his paralyzed leg. Part of the clot breaks off and travels to his lung, causing him extreme shortness of breath and the need for urgent hospitalization for a number of days. The shortness of breath happened suddenly in the middle of the day, and Joe thought he was going to die. As had been prearranged in such a situation, Joe managed to get to the phone and called a next-door neighbor, who was retired and who rushed over to help. Upon seeing Joe's distress, the neighbor decided that Joe needed an ambulance, which he called, using a list that had been placed by the phone. Then, as per plan, he called Joe's wife at work and then Joe's doctor. The neighbor then waited with Joe for the ambulance and accompanied him to the hospital.

Before she left work for the hospital, Joe's wife called her mother who had agreed to take the children should something like this happen. She would meet them after school and stay with them. From the second day on, they would stay at Joe's sister's home until things settled down at their own home; and so on.

The planning should not end with a coping scheme for the hospitalization, either. It is quite possible that the ill person will have greater limitations than before this crisis when he once again returns home. Thus, early in the hospitalization the spouse and the patient, if possible, or the spouse alone (or whoever the closest support person is) should arrange to meet with the physician and discuss the likely length of hospitalization and the expected status of the person when he/she is discharged. If new limitations are expected, it is important to discern as carefully as possible what these limitations will be and what sort of extra help or devices will be necessary to accommodate them. Then, the hospital social worker and discharge planner can be approached for help in organizing the additional needed services so that everything is in place when the person comes home. Will work schedules need to be adjusted to accommodate the new needs? Will more child care be necessary because the ill person can no longer contribute in this area? Will a hospital bed or commode need to be bought or rented? Will additional funds need to be found to pay for these things?

While it may be difficult to organize all this while one is trying to juggle the job, visiting at the hospital, and making sure there is time to spend with the kids, it is even harder to cope if such arrangements are delayed until after the person returns home.

If a family has a weak support system, this is much harder to do; but it is often possible to organize in advance services like childcare and other emotional and social supports that might be needed on an urgent basis. This might be done through a local chapter of an organization dealing with the particular illness involved (see Appendix 1), church groups, hospital services, or occasionally government offices.

By definition, emergencies take everyone by surprise, and even in the best of circumstances things may not run smoothly. Someone in a critical part of the plan may be out of town or ill. Thus, a couple of contingency plans should be worked out. A great benefit of working out a scheme for this sort of eventuality is that everyone feels more secure even if an emergency never occurs.

Because everyone is somewhat rattled in an emergency, it is important to write down critical information that might be forgotten in the heat of the moment. The following are a group of lists that, when available, can facilitate the handling of any unexpected situation:

◆ Keep, near the phone, a list of phone numbers of relatives and close friends who need to be called in an emergency. Make sure the list gives their responsibilities in an emergency. Give copies to each family member involved and to a close neighbor.

◆ Keep all emergency numbers: doctor, ambulance, hospital, police department, spouse's work number, children's school number, adult children's numbers, parent's numbers on a separate list by the phone.

◆ Keep a list of medications and a list of medical problems in your wallet. Make sure to include any peculiarities about your disease or any particular problems. Be sure to include allergies or other untoward reactions to drugs.

◆ Keep and wear a medical-alert bracelet or necklace that lists your diagnosis and allergies.

An ever-present thought for many families suffering chronic illness, is whether the ill person will die an early death. In some diseases, this may be a much more likely possibility than others. It is not morbid, shameful, or unlucky to think about this. It is normal, and rather than suppressing such concerns, family members should discuss and plan for this eventuality, even if it is distant. It is important to find out the wishes of the ill person in the event of death, to write wills, and to clarify the responsibilities of survivors. This may require legal consultation and documents, and is much better handled far in advance of one's death.

A chronically ill person often has silent concerns about his treatment, should he become terminally sick. These concerns should not remain confidential, but should be thoroughly discussed with close family members and with the doctor. An agreement should be reached about the extent of treatment in a clearly terminal situation. That is, the ill person should decide the extent to which he wishes to have artificial life support; if he wishes to avoid this, his feelings should be made clear to the family and doctor and, if appropriate, he may wish to draft a living will to formalize them. A living will is a document which states exactly to what extent you wish treatment to be pursued. It can also specifically state what you do not wish to be done. It states clearly whether you wish extraordinary means of life-support systems (heart and lung support systems) to be used and guides the family in making these decisions for you, should that become necessary.

♦ Medical crises are a dreaded possibility in families who are dealing with a chronic illness. Such crises can become quickly life threatening. The most important way to handle these fears is to set up a plan of action in case an emergency occurs.

♦ Make sure everyone who might be called upon in a crisis knows what is expected of them, and agrees to participate. Set up a contingency plan in case some of the principals are not available.

♦ While the ill person is still hospitalized, plan for and put in place changes in accommodation, assistance, and other needs that he/she will have when discharged.

◆ Keep lists of important phone numbers, medical diagnosis, medications, and other important information in readily accessible spots and in your wallet.

◆ Discussions about and plans for the ill person's possible death, even if it is not in the foreseeable future, can make the family and the person with the illness feel more secure about the family's future.

CHAPTER 5

Finding and Using
Community Resources

When an illness or disability is first diagnosed, there is a great deal of emotional upheaval and activity. But after the immediate crisis and when the person has achieved medical stability, the need to understand and gain information about the illness or disability and its implications for all aspects of the person's life, becomes of primary importance. It also becomes very important to locate and acquire the equipment and devices that will be needed to manage the changes due to the illness and disability, so that the person and his family can function as normally as possible.

To utilize optimally the resources that are available, it is first necessary to understand the purpose for and responsibilities of the professionals who work with the ill or disabled, and their families. Because many types of health-care professionals exist and offer similar, but different services, families may become confused about what is available and may not know how to evaluate and select the right services for their situation.

This chapter offers brief descriptions of some of the professions from which services might be accessed, suggests ways to locate these services, and lists some useful criteria for selecting appropriate professional help. We also include information about vocational rehabilitation services, devices, and equipment, as these services are so frequently helpful. This discussion will necessarily be but a brief introduction and is not intended to be comprehensive. Hopefully, it will make the reader aware of the sorts of things that exist and encourage him/her to look for more detailed information about services that seem potentially helpful.

To re-create as normal a life as possible in spite of the irrevocable changes of illness or disability, it is important to be informed, to ask questions, and to seek information. Libraries, home health agencies, organizations that certify health professionals, and illness-related organizations can be very informative about the various roles of professionals, selecting professionals, and about new equipment and available assistive devices.

When an ill or disabled person utilizes the services of an out-patient or inpatient rehabilitation program because of the loss of a body part, paralysis, or some loss of function, he/she will be served by a team of professionals. These people are trained to evaluate and plan treatment programs with patients to restore as much independence of functioning as possible, and provide whatever equipment and devices would help to reach that goal. Some of these professionals who are part of a rehabilitation team are below. (Descriptions of occupations are based on the U.S. Department of Labor, *Dictionary of Occupational Titles,* 4th edition, 1977, and *Community Health and Medical Guide,* 1987–1988, Westchester Region I, Health and Medical Guides, Inc., New York).

Physical Therapist: The physical therapist focuses on problems of mobility for accident victims, stroke victims, the handicapped, and others with injury or disease of the muscle, nerve, joint, or bone. Physical therapists also develop exercise programs for patients suffering cardiac and pulmonary disability. All aspects of mobility including, for example, transfer and ambulation, maintaining range of motion of extremities, how to use a wheelchair, or setting up an appropriate exercise program, are all part of the expertise of these professionals. They can recommend appropriate kinds of cushions or types of chairs or ambulation assistance devices. One of the goals of the physical therapist is to train or retrain the ill or disabled to perform as much as possible the activities they were able to perform prior to injury or illness, even if it is with assistive devices or in a new way. Also, physical therapy programs help to prevent increasing disability following a loss of body part, partial or total paralysis of a body part, or changes in the function of the body part due to disease (e.g., arthritis). The physical therapist develops both manual and non-manual exercises to improve or maintain muscle function, increase muscle strength and motor skills that will enable or increase ambulation, transfers, and daily living activities. Sometimes these functions can be improved to the point that a person previously needing assistance will be able to develop enough muscle strength to transfer from his/her bed to the wheelchair.

A person with arthritis, working with a physical therapist, might learn structured activities to maximize energy, put less stress on the joints, manage the pain, and learn how to pace activities. The physical therapist uses a variety of techniques and equipment. Heat, cold, massage, ultrasound, and electrical stimulation are often used as well as weights, mats, pulleys, and exercise machines, for example. In many areas, physical therapists will come to the home to continue activities that were begun in the hospital, since tailoring exercise programs, and fitting and adjusting assistive and supportive devices, as well as other aids, is best done with the person in his usual environment.

Occupational Therapist: The occupational therapist works with the patient and other members of the staff to develop devices and programs to help the ill or disabled achieve strength, coordination, and mobility, so that they can resume their own dressing, feeding, grooming, and cooking, etc.—activities that they did as part of normal daily routines before, and which will allow for independent living and renewed participation in previously enjoyed activities where possible. The occupational therapist will also plan programs to focus on activities, such as prevocational, vocational, and home-making skills, and activities of daily living, to prepare the ill or disabled for return to employment, assist in restoration of functions, and aid in adjustment to disability. The occupational therapist coordinates educational, recreational, and social activities designed to help patients regain physical functioning, or adjust to handicaps. They also design and construct special equipment for patients, and suggest adaptations of the patients work/living environment. It is part of the occupational therapist's job to be aware of what is available in the community, and what the latest equipment is to minimize the various disabilities, so that they can make recommendations, and order supplies and equipment. They also may design, make, and fit adaptive devices, such as splints and braces.

While in a rehabilitation setting or in the hospital, it is an opportune time to speak with the physical therapist and occupational therapist to assess what you may need at home. Occupational therapists as well as physical therapists can usually arrange home visits after discharge.

Medical Social Worker: The medical social worker helps patients and their families learn about and obtain maximum benefits from medical care. They provide individual and family counseling and utilize resources, such as family and community agencies, to assist patients in resuming life at home. While in the hospital, the social worker can assess the ill or disabled person's financial situation and make the necessary arrangements for the appropriate financial services, either from federal, state, or private insurance. They can also assist in finding appropriate housing or other resources like homemaking services, that might make the person's return to the community easier. Possibly the social workers most unique contribution comes from their training and knowledge about Medicaid, Medicare, and Social Security eligibility and how to apply, as well as their familiarity with community health agencies, independent living programs, federal and city programs, and other services needed by the ill or disabled. Social workers who are really interested and familar with what is out in the community and know how to access it, can speed up the process of obtaining resources because of their understanding of how the bureaucratic system works.

Speech Pathologists: Speech pathologists provide remediation for the loss of speech and language abilities due to illness, disability, stroke, or head injuries. They use a variety of communication devices: computers, pictorial devices, communication boards, esophageal speech, etc., to help restore as much communication ability as possible. For example, working with a person who has Lou

Gehrig's disease (amyotrophic lateral sclerosis), a speech pathologist would ascertain with the patient his/her energy level, desires, and ability level. Then, after an appropriate device is chosen to facilitate communication, the speech pathologist will teach the patient exercises to strengthen the necessary muscles as much as possible so that he/she can effectively use the device.

Speech pathologists also work with persons suffering speech impairment after strokes, head injuries, and removal or paralysis of the vocal cords. Many speech pathologists work in the community and in head injury centers. Because of the increasing survival of persons suffering severe head injury, there are head trauma programs in many cities that provide diagnosis, remediation, and management of cognitive and behavioral problems resulting from head trauma or stroke.

Dietitian: The dietitian can help educate patients and families, and plan menus for the proper diets, to help manage medical problems such as cardiovascular disease, diabetes, hypertension, high cholesterol, etc. Registered dietitians and certified nutritionists come to the home as part of a home health agency team, or work privately.

Sometimes it is only after discharge that the real needs of the family become apparent. Even if the rehabilitation team has evaluated the home prior to discharge, suggestions and changes made, and the equipment bought, one's ability to cope and function at home can be quite a different story from one's ability to function in the very accessible rehabilitation setting. The ill or disabled person can be doing very well in the hospital or rehabilitation program, but then when he is placed on his own in the home environment, the transition may be difficult, and symptoms can get worse.

If arrangements have not been made prior to discharge to have a public health nurse visit the home, these arrangements can be made through the physician after discharge. A registered visiting nurse from a public health agency will come to the home and assess the home environment. He/she will suggest changes in living arrangement and recommend assistive devices to adapt to the home environment, so it will be more comfortable and suited to the disabilities of the ill or injured person. These nurses are trained in finding ways to solve the problems that make it difficult to meet one's daily needs. They list the daily tasks that are not being properly accomplished, determine what the problems are, and make recommendations to solve them. They work with a team that includes nutritionists, occupational and physical therapists, speech therapists, social workers, and home health aides to provide resources and professionals who will help people adapt at home and make the most of their abilities despite their limitations.

When a public health nurse is called in, he/she will first do an evaluation. If the family is functioning well and needs nothing, she/he will not come back; but if it seems that there is a need for any one of the professionals on the team, the public health nurse will arrange for their visit, contact them, and handle the billing process. For example, a nurse might find that a person with emphysema has difficulty with his daily hygiene. After an evaluation of the person's needs and discussion with him, she can arrange for a home health aide to come into the home and help with personal care such as bathing. Visiting nurses can arrange for oxygen in the home, and they can arrange for visits by a respiratory therapist. Other ill or disabled persons might have special needs such as monitoring blood sugar, monitoring the side effects of new medication, changing dressings, and taking care of bed sores. The registered nurse can do these things, or teach the patient how to do them. Monitoring blood pressure and doing lab work can be done at home. They also can provide very specialized care and arrange for things such as home dialysis or the home administration of intravenous medications.

If necessary the nutritionist, also part of the team, can be called in to help patients requiring special diets plan proper meals to help manage their illnesses. Social workers are also available to provide counseling or help with Medicaid, Medicare, and insurance. The goal is to help the ill or disabled person to reach his/her potential within the disability and live as normal a life as possible.

Certified home health agencies can be found in the phone book under Home Health Agencies; discharge planners at the hospital can make referrals; also federal, county, or state Departments of Health are good sources for names of certified agencies. In Canada, contact the Ministry of Health or Public Health Department of Municipalities. Also, the library reference sections have books that list agencies and give descriptions of the particulars of each. The agencies will have differing fee scales. Some of the visiting nurse agencies are nonprofit, while others are operated on a for-profit basis. When contacting an agency, you should ask how they are operated. Some agencies adjust fees on a sliding scale according to the family's ability to pay. Most of the services that are needed qualify for reimbursement from Medicare, Medicaid, and health insurance. In Canada, some are covered under provincial health plans. What is not covered must be paid by the individual. Check both nonprofit and for-profit agencies to compare costs and eligibility. If you are interested in evaluation for services, contact an agency in your community and speak to your physician for a referral and recommendations.

After a period of adjustment at home, it may become clear that the family and the ill person have not been very successful in coping with their new life situation. Family members, the registered nurse, or other professionals may recognize that it is necessary and appropriate to arrange for psychological counseling. Once this decision has been made, it is necessary to find out what resources are available.

One of the most helpful sources of support is illness-specific associations. Nearly every serious long-term illness or injury has an association devoted to helping persons who suffer from that problem. In addition to a national organization, most of these associations, especially those representing the more common illnesses, have chapters servicing local communities as well as the states and provinces. We have listed many of them in Appendix 1. They are also listed in the phone book, usually under the type of illness represented, and in Community Health and Medical Guides. Most libraries carry in the reference section a comprehensive guide to all national associations. They also have books listing all provincial, state, county, and local community services. The reference librarian can easily retrieve these books for you.

The associations representing the various illnesses and disabilities provide the latest information on research, the names of professionals in the community who provide counseling, referrals to agencies for home care or nursing care, as well as their own home services, and educational classes. But probably the most important service they offer is the understanding of the problems a person faces, because their members have had the same experience and had to face the same problems. Almost all such associations offer numerous support services for the sufferers of that particular illness. For example, many branches of the National Multiple Sclerosis Society have a chapter services coordinator whose department provides telephone support groups, home visits, and referral to support groups in the community. The National Multiple Sclerosis Society also provides a great deal of literature on living with multiple sclerosis and family coping.

These associations may not be right for everyone, however. Some couples, individuals, or families who develop serious problems with communication, intimacy, or social interaction as the impact of the illness becomes more apparent may not be able to get the help they need through the illness-related organizations. The need for individual professional counseling may become apparent. If counseling services become necessary, it is important to know the various disciplines available and how to select the most appropriate counselor.

Psychologists: Psychologists are professionals who hold a doctorate (Ph.D., Psy.D., Ed.D.) and who are trained in prevention, diagnosis, and treatment of mental, emotional, and behavioral disorders. Psychologists employ a number of different techniques, such as behavior therapy (relaxation training, biofeedback), family therapy, psychodrama, and psychodynamic psychotherapy to assist people in adjusting to their life situations. Many psychologists specialize in the areas of rehabilitation psychology, illness and disability, and death and dying.

It is important that the psychologist you choose understands illness and disability, and the problems of coping peculiar to these problems. Psychologists are also licensed by the state in which they practice. If a psychologist is licensed, he/she is able to take third-party payments. Insurance policies that cover out-patient mental health will reimburse the patient for these services.

Psychiatrist: Psychiatrists are physicians who have specialized in the area of mental health. Psychiatrists are trained to diagnose and treat emotional, mental, and behavioral disorders, using a variety of psychotherapy techniques, and when indicated, prescribing medications. Like psychologists, clinical social workers, and other mental health professionals, some psychiatrists are interested and specialize in the area of physical illness and disability, or death and dying. Many psychiatrists are trained additionally in family therapy.

Clinical Social Worker: A clinical social worker is a professional who is trained to provide diagnosis, treatment, and prevention of mental and emotional disorders. A clinical social worker has been trained to do psychotherapy and provide treatment to individuals, couples, families, and groups. Social workers who have met the advance training requirements are members of the Academy of Certified Social Workers (A.C.S.W.). A clinical social worker with six or more years experience can receive insurance reimbursement.

Pastoral Counselor: Pastoral counselors are also available to provide psychotherapy services. There are many church-run counseling centers to provide individual, family, and group psychotherapy. Pastoral counselors usually have training and degrees in social work or psychology.

To locate a therapist, there are many sources of referral:

◆ Friends, family members, personal physician, and clergy.

◆ The American and Canadian Medical Associations, the American Psychological Association, the National Association of Social Workers (Appendix 1), or the county psychological and social work associations, as well as clinics and community mental health centers. The names of your county or local associations are listed in the phone book or are available at the local library in the reference section. The listings will include information about accessibility, eligibility, and fees.

◆ Illness-related organizations (Appendix 1) also can provide the names of professionals and agencies who then will be not only trained counselors but also knowledgeable about the specific illness or disability.

♦ Local family institutes that provide training and treatment can be very inexpensive and helpful. Look in the phone book under Family Therapy Institutes.

You might not know exactly what type of counseling you need. The following section might help you focus your search for a counselor a bit. Usually families who are coping with physical illness or disability will be having problems coping in one of these areas: bereavement and grieving issues, communication issues, sexual issues, personal issues related to how to handle certain things, and issues interfering with resuming work or interpersonal relationships. Families who are coping with physical illness or disability are not in need of psychoanalysis or interpersonal work to alter their character structure. There are specific feelings, thoughts, and ways of behaving that are relevant to the ill or disabled person, his/her children, spouse, and other significant relatives, and that are unique to coping with chronic illness or disability. A counselor is needed who will be able to bring these feelings to the surface, help the person and family recognize the appropriate feelings and the problems with communication and relationships within the family, and facilitate healthy adaptation. There are psychiatrists, psychologists, social workers, and pastoral counselors who have been trained in this area. Counselors specializing in this type of work understand these issues.

The following is a list of questions to take to a first visit (consultation) with a professional counselor. The counselor should not be defensive about answering these questions. If he/she is, this may not be the right counselor for you. Don't be afraid to ask the questions; your mental health may depend on the counselor you choose!

♦ What is your training or orientation? For example, do you use psychoanalysis, behavior therapy, interpersonal psychotherapy, family therapy?

- Are you currently seeing families or individuals who are dealing with issues related to illness or disability?

- Is the area of "death and dying" or "illness and disability" an area of interest or specialization for you?

- Are you knowledgeable and comfortable talking about the problems, emotions, and issues related to illness, death, and disability?

The family or family member should be able to feel comfortable about their choice and feel that the professional understands the particular issues that need to be discussed. Some professionals will not be comfortable or familiar with talking about death and illness. This you need to know before investing time and energy in an ill-fated therapeutic relationship. Make sure you feel comfortable and like talking to the professional you choose.

Another resource available in the community is the vocational rehabilitation services. Contact to initiate these services, which usually begin after discharge from the hospital or rehabilitation program is made through the medical social worker in the hospital. However, if such contact has been overlooked, it can be made after discharge through one's physician, a home health agency, or by calling the state vocational rehabilitation office nearest your community and asking them what is necessary for you to do to have an appointment. Career counselors are also available as part of agencies, or in private practice. Career counseling can provide valuable insight into one's abilities, interests, and career options.

State Divisions of Vocational Rehabilitation provide medical, psychological, and vocational evaluation. When necessary, many such offices supply psychotherapy, counseling, and guidance services. They also supply wheelchairs, artificial limbs, prosthetics, orthotics, and other assistive devices. Training in a college, trade or commercial school, and on-the-job training is also a possibility. Vocational rehabilitation services also include equipment and licenses for work on the job or in establishing a small business, placement assistance in a job, and placement follow-up, as well as many other services.

The *National Resource Directory: An Information Guide for*

Persons with Spinal Cord Injury and Other Physical Disabilities contains a listing of state vocational rehabilitation agencies and a description of services provided by them. It is an excellent source of information on available services and programs for persons whose mobility has been affected by illness or injury. (See Appendix 2.)

Some states have Personal Care Attendants Programs for employed or employable people who meet certain financial and other criteria. The *National Resource Directory,* mentioned above, provides further information about these programs. Some communities provide government-assisted transportation to and from work, or shopping for the disabled. One such program is the Wheel Trans program in Toronto. By getting in touch with community government departments and organizations that service the handicapped, one can obtain information about available services. Counseling services may also be available through these same sources.

Assistance for persons with a disability is not limited to community services, either. Many types of special equipment are available to assist with almost any type of physical limitation. For example, a number of adaptive devices are provided by the telephone companies for persons who are blind, deaf, or suffer with physical impairment. Speaker phones, card dialers, and head sets can allow people with no use of their hands or arms to use the telephone independently. There are also voice-keyed electric typewriters, automatically operated page turners, environmental control units, electronic feeders, computer systems, various electronic and mechanical devices, as well as special clothing. Biomedical Engineering Centers provide assistance to persons in need of adaptive devices to make their home or job more accessible. These centers specialize in designing or recommending equipment to meet specific needs at home or on the job. (See Appendix 1 and *National Resource Directory,* Editor Barry Corbet, National Spinal Cord Injury Association: Mass., 1985.)

Products for anxiety management (relaxation training tapes, anxiety reduction tapes) are available to make life easier, and to help make it possible to do things independently again. Page turners, jar openers, and a variety of products to enable hand and leg mobility are available from medical-surgical pharmacies or medical supply retailers. Most of what is available is listed in the *Spinal Network* and the *National Resource Directory* (see Appendix 2), and is valuable for any type of physical disability or illness-related disability. Also illness-related associations and home health agencies, as well as physicians, occupational, and physical therapists, are aware of what is being invented and can help you order it.

◆ Libraries, home health agencies, organizations that certify health professionals, and illness-related organizations can be very informative about community agencies, the various roles of professionals, how to select professionals, about new equipment, and available assistive devices.

◆ A registered public health nurse from a public health agency can come to your home to evaluate the environment, make recommendations for equipment and services, and bring in a team of professionals to provide needed services. Arrangements for these services can be made through your physician at your request.

◆ Psychotherapists knowledgeable about illness and disability will be able to understand the specific issues and work effectively with the family. Families and individuals in the family who are coping with physical illness and disability are not usually in need of psychoanalysis. The focus needs to be on the changes that have taken place in relationships and communication within the family, as well as the impact of the illness or disability on the ill or disabled person, and on each member of the family.

TWO

Emotional Stresses on the Individual and Family

◆ ──────────────── ◆

CHAPTER 6

Answering "Why Me?"

Why me? Why us? Why our family? Why did God choose us for this misfortune? What have we done to deserve this? Do not all these questions pass through the minds of the victims of serious illness or injury, and their family members? They are, of course, unanswerable questions. But failing to realize and admit that there are no answers may keep us from moving beyond the initial shock of our unwelcome fate to the eventual adaptation to it. In this chapter, we will present three family situations in which the members grapple with the question of Why me? or Why us? The first family is a young family with preteenage children. A disabling stroke might, in part, be the result of the victim's failure to take prescribed medication, and this introduces the confounding factor of guilt. The second family, Douglas and Susan, is a retirement-age couple who have eagerly anticipated this time in their lives, and now it is marred by a progressive illness. The final vignette is of a carefree young couple, both of whom sustain severe permanent injury in a motor vehicle accident.

Each of these family units deals with different aspects of this issue. We will present different family members' experiences of the "Why?" question and suggest ways in which they can adapt and cope.

Neil and Joy

◆ Neil and Joy, ages thirty-five and thirty-three, were married twelve years and had three preteenage children. Neil, who was an auto mechanic, had been hypertensive and on medication since age thirty. He did not like to take pills, though, and frequently forgot them. He had also been advised to have his blood pressure checked every month, but because he felt perfectly well, he rarely found time to have this done. Joy was concerned about this and, at first, reminded him almost daily about taking the pills. This annoyed Neil, and Joy soon quit nagging him because it was not worth the tension it caused. Anyway, she had to agree that he did seem perfectly healthy.

One day at work, Neil suffered a stroke and lost the use of his left arm and leg. In the hospital over the next few days, he regained very little strength. Then his doctor recommended a rehabilitation program to teach him to walk with a walker. Neil suddenly realized he would never walk normally again. He picked up his blood pressure pills from the bedside table and threw them across the hospital room. After throwing the pills, he sat down on the bed and wept. He felt like a total failure. Why hadn't he taken his medication? He felt he had caused this terrible stroke.

When one first learns he has a chronic or debilitating illness, it is not uncommon for the person to feel guilty and responsible for the consequences of the illness. When there is the possibility, as in this example, that following medical advice more closely might have prevented some of the devastating consequences that ensued, the inital reaction can be quite painful. This sort of feeling and the inability to cope with it can result in violent displays of temper and tears. A person who had difficulty accepting the need to take medication (an expression perhaps of his denial of his medical problem) may have a difficult time coping with his guilt and may benefit from brief, professional counseling. Whether or not the person could have avoided his current situation is irrelevant at this point; both he and other members of the family need to recognize and accept this before they will be able to move on. Excessive self-blame may lead to deep depression and may produce severe tension in the family. Family members, to be helpful, have to step back and be sympathetic. The person feels guilt and remorse because he certainly did not want to harm himself; he may even feel worse for his family members because of the pain he may have caused them.

Some people approach this sort of misfortune quite differently. They are able to find a degree of comfort in being able to answer, at least in part, the nagging question, "Why me?" At least the person in this position can hold himself accountable, and there is no ambiguity about it. As long as the person does not feel excessive guilt or a need to be punished, he may find the belief that he is responsible, tolerable and helpful in allowing him to move on with his life. He will be able to adapt to the changes and reestablish a satisfying life for himself.

◆ Neil entered a rehabilitation program and remained in the hospital for several weeks. He found it difficult to attend his rehabilitation sessions and often did not get up to go. Joy would visit him every night. He waited all day long for her visit. Then one night she walked in, and before she even greeted or kissed him, she said accusingly, "Why haven't you been going to your rehabilitation sessions? How are you ever going to be able to do anything if you just lay there in bed all day?" This precipitated a major argument, which resulted in both Neil and Joy saying things they wished they had not. Joy was surprised by her own anger, which startled her in its intensity. Neil felt he deserved Joy's anger.

Neil's guilt about not taking his medication and his excessive self-blame may be behind his lack of motivation to participate in his own rehabilitation. The way in which people react to the news of illness is in part related to their ways of coping with life stressors and illness, prior to the current illness. If Neil's style of coping with problems prior to the stroke was to avoid or deny unpleasantness, then he will use that style of coping now. His way of coping, though, has been complicated by the inevitable question "Why has this happened to me?" Unfortunately, in this example, both Neil and Joy are finding the same answer. That is, that Neil is to blame because he did not take his medication. The guilt and hurt this thought causes Joy is reflected in her lack of sympathy and her anger at Neil. It is possible and frequently unavoidable (although not an acceptable feeling to the person feeling it), that the well spouse will blame the ill person for bringing this disaster upon themselves and the family; at the same time, this well spouse also feels self-blame, because she fears that maybe she did not do enough to prevent this from happening. Joy's guilty feelings result from a memory of a night when she had been too tired to push and argue about his taking the medications and had found herself thinking, on that particularly bad night, that she wished her argumentative and stubborn husband would get sick, and then he would wish he had listened.

Searching to find out why the illness or injury has struck them helps some families gain a sense of control, and gives life a sense of order and meaning again. It is their attempt to make something unreasonable and unexplainable, reasonable and explainable. However, while it is normal and common to search for reasons why the disaster befell them, it is rare that they find satisfying answers, since there are usually no certain or clear-cut answers. Sometimes the afflicted person or family members blame God, and then feel guilty and frightened at their sacrilege. Other times, they blame themselves or other family members, hoping to understand and avoid feeling guilty. There is often a pervasive rage at one's bad luck. Like Shakespeare's Hamlet, the ill person cries out in pain against the "slings and arrows of outrageous fortune."

Veiled accusations and self-guilt can only be expected to elicit angry responses from a spouse or other relatives; this is true especially in the setting where he/she already feels responsible. This tacit blaming and counter-blaming can escalate and continue for long periods. Joy's concern about Neil recovering and her own reactions to his illness prevent her from thinking through ways to help Neil cope with his guilt and participate in his rehabilitation. Because of her own pain and grief, she fails to see that Neil is not just being stubborn or obstinate; he is suffering deeply as well.

Joy needs a strategy to help Neil. First, Joy must get her feelings out in the open. If she has a close girlfriend, a family member like a sister, or a clergyman, counselor, or doctor, who would be nonjudgmental, she should arrange to meet with him/her just to vent her feelings. She needs to talk about her feelings of rage and guilt with someone who will just listen and not react emotionally and negatively. Then she can begin to put these feelings in perspective and begin to adjust to her new life situation.

The next step is for Joy to talk with close friends, other family members, or even a professional counselor about Neil's reaction. Getting the family's advice and participation in this should pave the way for him to begin adjusting and coping. Family members could attend rehabilitation sessions with Neil, encouraging him and keeping him company. Future plans must be discussed with Neil. This is necessary not only because he is central to those plans, but also because it shows him that he is still needed and will be depended upon. Seeking his advice and complaining about not having his help with activities he used to help with at home will also give him the message that he continues to be important. Children, other family members, and friends can play critical roles by finding ways of letting Neil know he is still an important part of their lives. His children asking him to help with a math assignment or attend a school concert, his wife asking him how to fix things he used to fix, and friends hiring him to do some jobs for them, are all specific ways the family and friends can be helpful.

It is not useful or healthy for a couple to focus on what is not changeable. By changing his approach to his health and realizing he is still an integral part of the family, Neil can help to ensure the most satisfying—though different—future possible for himself and Joy. The danger of focusing on medication that was not taken in the past or mistakes that were made, is that the entire family can give up responsibility for the present (not going to rehabilitation sessions, for example) and jeopardize their future.

◆ After she left the hospital, Joy felt very badly about her argument with Neil. When she reached the house, she ran to their bedroom and broke into uncontrollable sobs. "My life is ending, my life is ending," she heard herself saying over and over.

This is a crisis period for the whole family. The spouse is often forgotten in the chaos surrounding the onset of a major health problem; yet the spouse is almost always frightened and is often in a state of panic. He/she may be angry and perplexed by the sudden catastrophic event in their young lives, or may feel cheated and unlucky. These are painful feelings that result in sadness and frustration.

A couple in this situation has a very important task to accomplish. Together they need to come to an understanding that it is useless to blame themselves or each other for the illness. Any responsibility lies in the past, and what is now important is that they regain some control of future events. To do this they must begin to make good decisions together and plan activities for the future. Many activities and plans for the future can be made with Neil, but to do this it is necessary that both partners be good listeners. Joy and Neil need the opportunity to express these feelings to each other without feeling that their partner is being judgmental. This can best be done if one partner just talks for a few minutes, and the other listens without interrupting; then the roles can reverse, and the listener can become the talker. Each may be amazed at what the other is thinking; often if a couple has had a good pre-illness relationship, this type of conversation will allow conciliation and a return of closeness. If they did not communicate well pre-illness, this will be much more difficult and may require the mediation of a third party, usually someone not close to the couple, like a clergyman, social worker, or other professional.

◆ When Neil came home from the hospital, the children, especially Michael, his ten-year-old son, were ecstatic. But over the next few days, Michael realized his dad wasn't the same dad anymore. He would not play hockey with him; they could not ride bicycles together; nothing was the same. He did not even seem to like to talk to Michael. It made Michael feel like crying; he wished for a new dad. He prayed for God to give him back his old dad. Had he done something wrong for God to cause this to happen to him?

A preteenage child is very susceptible to feeling responsible for the illness of a parent and the inevitable changes in the family. He does not understand what has happened and is frightened that things will never be normal again, and that he might lose the parent altogether. He wants to feel his family is under control and wants to find a way to make things better again. He will mourn the loss of his relationship with his father and feel angry about the changes. These feelings are confusing and disturbing. Reassuring children that no one is responsible for the illness is important.

In searching out why this has happened, many children and teens blame themselves. It is very important to spend time talking alone with each of the children. They should be asked how they feel about what has happened, and their feelings acknowledged. For instance, if a ten-year-old child says, "I am mad at Daddy for doing this because he can't play hockey with me anymore," it would only make the child feel guilty to respond, "How can you say such a thing when you know your father didn't do this on purpose." It would be more beneficial to the child in helping him adjust to his own scary feelings and his father's disability by saying, "I know you feel upset at Dad, and it is OK to feel that way. It is true that he can't play hockey anymore, but I bet we can find a whole lot of things he can do with you. And since he won't be spending so much time at work, he will be able to spend more time with you now." Even when they do not bring it up in conversation, it is important to assure children that they did nothing to cause any of the changes in their family. This was not the result of their making their ill parent angry in the past, or the result of any bad thoughts they might have had about their ill parent in the past. It is important to tell children what is going on and what is being discussed with respect to future plans. Let them discuss their feelings about it all. If they have questions, they need to know that they can ask those questions and get true answers. To answer children's questions, just give them the information they are asking about and not long explanations. Children need to know what they are curious about, but too elaborate explanations can be confusing. "Why can't Daddy play hockey anymore?" "Daddy has had a heart attack and his heart isn't as strong as it used to be, so he can't run as much as he used to" is adequate. You do not need to go into a long explanation of the reason for the heart attack, or frighten them by saying that hockey might cause another heart attack. Observe children's behavior at these times as well. Many times children blame themselves for a parent's illness or disability. They unconsciously think they are responsible. One way this shows itself, is that the child becomes exceedingly helpful and good. If you notice that your child is acting unusually well behaved and trying to be very good both at home and at school, talk to them about the possibility that they may be blaming themselves. Ask them what they are thinking and feeling. Reassure them, even if they don't say they are blaming themselves, that they are not to blame. Discuss with them what causes illnesses, and how it may have happened that their parent is sick or disabled. This kind of information also relieves children's fears that they may catch the illness themselves. This is a frequently unexpressed fear that children experience. Sometimes it makes things so much easier when a child is very good, especially when you're trying to manage the household with a newly diagnosed or disabled person, that it is easy to just accept it. But such behavior is not healthy, and children need to be relieved of such a heavy burden of responsibility.

Wait for children to ask about outcomes before explaining all the possible consequences of the illness. Children like to be helpful, and if there are ways they can be, they should be allowed to help. They can do chores around the house, run errands, etc. It is necessary for parents to show the children that although things are different, relationships with the ill parent and as a family will continue. Trips can be planned together, and community activities attended together. The children need to know that the ill parent will still participate in their lives in some fashion, even if it now means playing checkers and watching TV instead of playing hockey.

The important thing for children is usually knowing that the parent is there and wants to spend time with them in whatever fashion; the fact that the parent can no longer participate in very active sports may be of much more importance to the parent than the child. Optimistic and realistic planning of family outings and activities demonstrate that the family can continue to function as before.

Douglas and Susan

◆ Douglas and Susan were both in their late fifties when Douglas began to notice that Susan was forgetting things that they had

BUILDING A NEW DREAM

discussed in day-to-day conversations. At first he did not think much about it, but he knew there was a real problem the day Susan's friend, Ellen, called to tell Douglas that Susan had been by for coffee and could not find her way home.

Douglas had been planning for his retirement for years. He had built up a good pension and had risen to an executive position in the pharmaceutical firm he worked for. He and Susan—there weren't any children—had given up many things to save for retirement. He saw his plans crumbling before his eyes. Not only could she not participate in their many plans; he could hardly have an adult conversation with her anymore. Had he done something bad or wrong to deserve this? He had worked so hard all his life and had so many plans and now they were all falling apart! Then he remembered. Once, about fifteen years ago, shortly after it had become clear that Douglas and Susan would never have children and both were terribly disappointed, Douglas had met a young woman at a company conference and had spent the weekend with her. Douglas was a very religious and God-fearing man. Maybe this was God's way of punishing him.

Alzheimer's Disease, or memory loss, has struck this couple just as they are reaching the time in life when they hoped to sit back and relax, and reap the rewards of many long years of work. It is important that whenever an elderly person begins to show signs of dementia that he/she be seen by a physician before it is assumed they have a disease like Alzheimer's. Since some causes of dementia are remediable, it is extremely important that those be excluded as possibilities.

Many progressive diseases strike at this time in life, and it is very difficult because it is a time when people are about to let go of work. The shock and disappointment need some explanation to be bearable. It is natural to search to understand why you have been the one to suffer this fate. At such times, it is common to think that something one did caused the misfortune, particularly if the person who is suffering is someone who takes a lot of responsibility for the way things have turned out in his life.

In this example, Douglas's belief that his one-time affair has now brought upon him this misfortune, is one way for him to comprehend such poor luck. It is an indication of how devastated he feels. Dwelling on past events as reasons for present misfortunes is often a warning sign that a person is having difficulty mourning what is lost and moving on to readjusting to whatever the new reality is. Feelings of "Why me, why us?" are almost universal in situations of severe illness, accident, or loss of life. It is unanswerable and a part of the mourning process. When it is no longer a central question or controlling thought, this is a sign that the person or family is moving on to healing, acceptance, and readjustment.

When a person is mourning but progressing, these thoughts do not haunt him/her. However, if these thoughts are persistent or if they prevent progress in returning to activities, then they need to be addressed either with the family, or with one's physician, or some appropriate health-care professional. Douglas needs to tell his physician or clergy that he believes this has happened to him because of his affair. His belief that his affair caused him to be punished is based on his wish that everything in life was controllable. Douglas looks for a reason for his misfortune because he needs to feel he has control over his life. It is more disturbing to some people to think that they do not have absolute control over their destiny, than to feel guilt about causing their misfortune. It will help him to hear reassurances and to learn that life is unpredictable. We have only so much control over our lives. While we can control many things, we are all subject to good or bad luck. By discussing these things, Douglas can reevaluate his situation and become less anxious and concerned about control.

◆ Over the next three years, things went from bad to worse with Susan. Douglas could no longer leave her by herself. He spoke to her like a child; it was almost as if now, in his long-awaited retirement, he was being saddled with the responsibility of a child, a responsibility which ironically he and Susan had been denied when they had so desired it many years ago. Except for an occasional afternoon at the golf course, Douglas spent all his time caring for Susan. He felt as if he were being smothered.

Probably the most difficult type of chronic illness with which to cope is an ongoing, progressive disease. Just as the family becomes adjusted to one phase of the illness, an exacerbation occurs and readjustment is necessary, and this brings new insecurities and uncertainty about the future. When one has a disease which stabilizes early, it can be much easier to resolve feelings of guilt and blame, and then life can return to some level of stability. With continually worsening disability, the patient or other family members can experience what feels like continual punishment and feelings of being trapped. Also, the continuing progression of the disease brings a steady stream of new losses to mourn. Grief is a constant companion.

In this example, Douglas has become isolated and unable to focus on his own needs. When this happens, the help of family members or close friends is necessary. Douglas needs to bring others in to give him a break; he and they need to map out a plan for taking turns to help with Susan's care. He would then have a better chance to find ways to handle his wife's needs without emotionally exhausting himself. (See Chapter 10: Preventing Emotional Exhaustion.) If this cannot be done, Douglas may suffer severe burnout. And if that happened, he might not be able to cope with her at all.

When there are no family or friends who are able to help, outside organizations might be able to give some respite assistance. Organizations like Visiting Nurses can be very helpful in this way. They can coordinate multidisciplinary services for the patient, provide specialized care, and arrange for outside caregivers for certain periods of time so that family members can have some time to themselves. Outside counseling or support groups run by illness-related associations—in this case the Alzheimer Association or Alzheimer Society—often help relatives get through the mourning process, help them recognize the sadness and anger they feel, and help them plan for ways to get aid in the caretaking. Some of these organizations even have telephone numbers where people can call and get advice or counseling over the phone in a crisis situation.

One way to help prevent constant mourning in the face of a

progressive illness like Alzheimer's disease or other neurologic illnesses is to get as much information as possible about the likely course of the disease from one's physician and from others with the same disease. This can give family members a picture of the likely future so they are forewarned, and, if necessary, can make preparations. (See Chapter 9: Managing Personality Changes, Bonita.)

Sam and Jody

◆ Their friends had always thought it fitting that Sam and Jody met at an off-road vehicle race. Both had loved motorcycles, sky diving, and other dangerous sports; they liked living on the edge. Both in their early twenties, the two spent almost all their free time participating in cycle-jumping competitions, and other daring activities. They were admired by many of their friends because of their carefree life-style. Sam's and Jody's charmed existence came to an abrupt end on a rainy day in May. They were both on Sam's motorcycle on a rainslick freeway when the back wheel slipped, throwing Sam over the handlebars and breaking his neck. Jody was trapped under the cycle, and her left leg was mangled and required amputation.

In the weeks that followed the accident, Sam began to realize and accept the devastation of his accident; he had always felt that he had no real control over his ultimate destiny, and when his number came up, that would be it. It was just his bad luck that his number had come up so early in the prime of his life.

Sam's mother felt quite differently. She was a widow and Sam was her only son. She had always worried about the danger her son courted and had cautioned him and even nagged him repeatedly about being more careful. Now she felt as if her worst fears were realized, and it was all his fault; not only had he destroyed his life and all her dreams for his future, he had destroyed her life as well. Maybe she should have done something else to prevent him from doing those dangerous things. If she hadn't countersigned the loan for his motorcycle, would he be OK today?

There are many different ways people cope with disease and disability sustained by injury. One way is to externalize and blame their misfortune on bad luck as Sam has done in this example. This attitude may help Sam cope with some very painful feelings and sadness. As long as Sam's way of coping does not lead to his giving up on his life and withdrawing into a shell, this attempt to gain mastery and control may work for some time. The danger is that Sam is not experiencing the expected and normal amount of sadness, and may become embroiled in a power struggle with his mother as a result of their different ways of coping and reacting.

Sam's mother is engaging in self-blame and guilt. The belief that one is totally responsible for all that can happen in this lifetime does not allow for unknowns and chance events in life or fate. Neither a fatalistic view that one has no control over one's life and that all the unfortunate things that happen are the result of bad luck, nor the equally rigid view that nothing but one's own behavior affects one's life, is a very functional philosophy in helping one to cope with catastrophic illness and injury. To adjust in these circumstances, one needs to adopt an approach that is flexible enough for a good balance and will enhance the opportunity to live one's life to the fullest after the initial recovery. Many people manage to adapt without excessive guilt or blame. When there is difficulty, it might be the result of too rigid a view either way. When this is the case, talking with a health-care professional or clergy to help bring some balance to a highly rigid view can be helpful. Though sadness is appropriate, excessive blame leads to self-defeating behavior. The goal is to reach a point where there is sadness without excessive self-denigrating blame, especially when this type of blame is preventing rehabilitation and adjustment.

◆ Jody's injury was less severe physically than Sam's. She would be able to be fitted with an artificial leg and would walk. However, in many ways, the injury was more devastating. She had known about the dangers of riding fast on rainslick highways, and in the corner of her mind she had some reservations about it, but she had made the decision to go along with it. For the rest of her life she would have to live with that decision; her plans for a career as an airline stewardess were shattered. But it was her fault; she had failed, and she would have to live with it.

Jody's response demonstrates a more adaptive style. While there is a danger of her blaming herself too much, she seems to be able to see what part her behavior played in what happened to her. It is important to learn about ourselves—to develop insight into our behavior—despite the pain these truths may bring. To gain insight into one's own actions, even one's day-to-day life, it is useful to sit down alone and ask "Why did I do what I did today," or "Why did I get angry at my children for seemingly no reason today?", and then try to answer these questions.

One has to be able to grow and learn even in the midst of tragedy. If Jody can successfully mourn her losses and feel the sadness and pain, while understanding that she did take risks and did affect the odds against herself, she has a good chance of participating in her recovery in such a way that she can cope and adjust to the consequences of her actions. This means that she would be able to find successful new career goals and have relationships that bring her a sense of happiness and feelings of being important to someone who is important to her. Jody may be able to learn from this experience what motivated her to take such chances, and from this point on, be more in a position to use her creativity and energy in more positive ways.

Our individual beliefs about why things that are bad happen become the way in which we understand why these devastations happen to us. Certain styles of coping and certain beliefs are more useful than others for adapting to and continually adjusting to the changes caused by illnesses and disabilities. For many people, religious beliefs help sustain them through times of tragedy. Many religious and nonreligious people believe that there is an overall plan to things. When illness or disability strike, it is understood to be God's will, and the reasons for it known only to God. Their faith and belief that there is a reason for all things, even if it is not clear at the moment, help families get through the painful self-searching, "Why me?" period of adaptation. Many people also have a belief and faith that things will get better. It can help further to speak with clergy for support and encouragement.

♦ Spouses are often as devastated by illness as the victim and experience many of the same feelings of guilt, loss, and sadness. Couples need to talk to each other about these feelings.

♦ Children may feel responsible for a parent's illness or disability, believing it is a result of something bad that they have done. Tell children what is going on, answer honestly questions they have, and encourage them to express their concerns and feelings.

♦ Feelings of "Why me?" or "Why us?" are really unanswerable and are part of the normal mourning process.

♦ When the question "Why me?" is no longer a constant thought, it is a sign of progress toward feeling sad without excessive self-blame or loss of faith in life.

♦ There are many different styles of coping and no one right way. The only thing of importance is that a person's coping style allows them to come to adjust to their changed circumstances.

♦ Guilt, self-blame, and accusations are common when illness strikes. It is important to recognize that these feelings really mask the sadness and helplessness one is feeling.

CHAPTER 7

Coping with Depression

The emotional impact of an illness is never limited to the person who has the illness. Every member of the family will in some way be touched by the problem and will experience some sort of emotional upheaval because of it.

Most often, feelings will be those of sadness and discouragement. This may be considered a form of depression and is an emotional response that is appropriate and common in the setting of chronic illness or disability. The concept of depression has been widely used by health professionals and lay people to describe a variety of moods as diverse as a day of sadness to a week of not getting out of bed all day. Because of this, we are often confused about what depression really is. To complicate the matter even further, it is often difficult to find a word or words that really describe feelings and emotional reactions. Therefore, our individual concepts of depression can range from the feeling that it is a frightening mental state that we would rather not admit, to the feeling that it is an overused emotion that is not taken seriously.

It is important to be able to distinguish between mild and severe depression, so that if an ill or disabled person or a member of the family shows signs that his emotional reactions have become so severe that he needs medication or professional counseling, these services can be sought. Feeling that one is out of control, helpless, and frightened can lead to feelings of despair. When despair and disillusionment become so prominent that the family is no longer functioning, the feelings are out of control and help is needed.

In this chapter, we will try to point out differences between mild and severe depression, and present hypothetical situations illustrating these to help you recognize and distinguish them. We will also talk about times and circumstances when family members and the ill or disabled person are more at risk to feel depressed. For those less severe depressions that do not require professional help, we will outline positive steps to take to relieve and modify those feelings. The first step is to identify normal or acceptable reactions to a given problem.

Sadness, loss of appetite, crying, anger, and sleeplessness after a serious chronic illness, terminal illness, or physical disability are *appropriate* normal responses to a major life stress. Family members as well as the ill or disabled person will find themselves crying and feeling very sad and discouraged. This is grieving.

Many people think one grieves only after a death. However, that is not true. Grieving is a common response to many types of loss. Included are those losses associated with chronic illness and disability, which can be pervasive and shattering. In fact, families may notice that when an ill person dies, they are not as sad as they were often before the death. Family members sometimes even feel relieved. That is because the family members have already mourned, long before the person's death, the losses of roles, dreams, plans, and life changes that the illness caused.

Grief is episodic for people with progressively debilitating illnesses that do not stabilize or stabilize only temporarily. During periods of stability, family members become more optimistic; but when things worsen, anger, disappointment, and sadness return. This sort of emotional roller coaster is particularly difficult, but becomes a fact of life for the family dealing with a progressively impairing illness or disability.

Grief usually does not become a serious depression requiring professional psychiatric care, though the symptoms can mimic such a condition. Because of the similarity of symptoms between the two conditions, it is important to differentiate them. For example, a person who is demoralized since learning of a diagnosis of a serious illness or after a disabling accident can react with symptoms also descriptive of a serious depression. He or she may be angry, feel worthless, withdraw, lose interest in previously enjoyed activities, have suicidal thoughts, feel inconsolable misery or fatigue, lose appetite, develop insomnia, headaches, backaches, upset stomachs, or constipation, and lose or gain weight. All these can also be symptoms of a serious depression as well as of grief.

However, there are differences. A seriously depressed person who cannot sleep will get up and worry about everything and anything. He will just feel nervous and jittery. A grieving person with a new diagnosis who can't sleep will get up and worry too, but he will worry about the course and consequences of the illness. Often, if one explores the symptoms of a grieving person, the reasons for them can be related to the illness or accident, unlike those of the severely depressed person who is not medically ill. For example, when an ill or disabled person loses interest in sex (a symptom associated with depressive illness also), it may be due to the illness itself, concerns about capability as a result of the illness, or the effects of a medication. It is not, as with depressive illness, a symptom of the depression and a consequence of depression. Severely depressed persons evaluate themselves, the world, and their future negatively and very critically; the ill or disabled person, on the other hand, is critical to the extent that it relates to the illness or disability and his feelings about the effects of the illness or disability on his life and family. These fears and fantasies are usually about the future and how it will now be changed.

Apathy is also part of feeling sad and discouraged. Apathy after a major illness is not serious depression. Apathy is part of the normal grieving process, which can come and go periodically. It is most likely but not necessary that feelings of sadness and loss will periodically return. Why shouldn't they? There have been great disappointments and changes; dreams have been shattered; roles permanently changed, and losses never to be regained.

But these feelings can exist while one carries out new and old life plans, works, socializes, and expresses love and affection. They are not mutually exclusive. It is only when they get in the way of and prevent good family relationships, impair productivity, stifle rehabilitation efforts, and prevent participation in and enjoyment of activities, that it is a problem.

Most symptoms of grief will not seriously endanger the well being of the grieving person. However, at times, mild normal depressions can become severe depressions. If symptoms like weight loss, sleep disturbance, suicidal thoughts, and headaches last a long time—more than eight weeks—and do not seem to be getting better, it may be that the reactions to the illness or disability have reached a point that outside help with the grieving process would be useful.

Other responses to the physical effects and life changes of an illness that may signal a more serious depression are these: The sadness never lifts, even momentarily. The person is repetitive about how awful he feels, repeating over and over again the same things; he is unable to ever smile or laugh. The guilt is unrelenting, or the external blaming continuous or, on the other hand, he is unable to express any emotion. He does not ever cry, but his affect is strained, and he is unable to function, go to work, or get up in the morning. Nothing makes a difference to him. No amount of talking helps.

This is the time to get outside help, because the grieving process and/or some medical condition has caused the grief to escalate to either a major affective (depressive psychiatric) disorder, or to some complicating medical problem. Evaluation of both possibilities needs to be done to determine what is causing the dysfunctioning and to offer treatment. Medical illnesses, medication, and changes in body chemistry due to illness or medication can also cause depression. Weight loss, for example, can occur as the result of catabolic changes, or as the result of medications that take away appetite. When symptoms become so severe and last over eight weeks, it is important to get a professional opinion about what it is that is happening.

At other times, there are no physical changes, but behavioral changes become severe. When a family member has a personality change so that he is always angry and sits all day watching television, withdrawing and complaining, family members need to be alert to the possibility that something more than grief may be occurring.

It is important to remember that requiring professional help does not mean that the grieving family member or ill person has developed a mental illness. Nor is it the same as when a person requires antidepressant therapy because of depressive illness or personality traits that cause him to continually express unhappiness, pessimism, or negativity about himself, the present, and the future. Responses to illness and disability, on the other hand, that include sadness, crying, unhappiness, and discouragement are expected and normal responses to loss, disappointment, fear, and change. These feelings can get out of hand because of the person's response to a devastating set of circumstances.

The following are some vignettes that illustrate the points we have been discussing.

◆ After the diagnosis of Hodgkin's Disease, and with the fatigue and nausea caused by the chemotherapy, Ann had been mourning the losses she felt, by crying and refusing to go on family outings. Her family left her alone, understanding how sad she was and feeling sad themselves. However, recently if anyone spoke to Ann she would explode, yelling and telling them to get out of her room. This was not like her. In addition, one morning, she refused to get out of bed and go to work. She was a clinical social worker and loved her career. Her mother became especially concerned when no matter what she said, Ann would not stop worrying each time she would try to leave the house to go grocery shopping. The final blow came one Sunday when Ann told her parents that she had decided life was not worth living as a result of her cancer, and that she could find no reason to go on. She felt so terrible inside that she just wanted to escape those feelings. She sat all day staring straight ahead and complaining how sick she felt. That night her mother could hear her walking around the house. Ann was fatigued, anxious, and hopeless. Her family had never seen their normally enthusiastic and optimistic daughter like this before.

Ann presents a picture that calls for professional help to help with the mourning process. Medication and/or psychotherapy can be very helpful if the grief has escalated to a major affective disorder as appears to be true in this case. Often there is unnecessary guilt or self-blame that is the reason the grieving has become a major depression. For some people, their self-image and sense of manliness or femininity is so shaken, or the feelings of isolation and of being different is so great, that they do not feel adequate to meet the tasks of living. This terrible sense of inadequacy leads to the debilitating levels of depression. With proper professional help, the size of the sadness can be reduced to manageable and appropriate proportions. For some people this can happen rapidly; for others more gradually over the course of a year or two. Sometimes medication is necessary.

Psychiatrists, psychologists, social workers, visiting nurses, or clergy can be very helpful when depression has become severe. In addition, when the severe symptoms of depression follow severe illness or disability, often results through therapy are very good. If you are concerned that a family member or the ill or disabled person has become severely depressed, ask a visiting nurse, doctor, or mental-health professional to assess the person.

◆ Nothing seemed important to George anymore. He sat all day anxiously waiting for his wife to come home. He could not concentrate on the television and the feelings inside were so terrible, he wished they would go away. At night he couldn't sleep, but he was tired. It was hard to move. He sat rigidly watching the front door. George was so afraid. He did not want his family to think he was now, in addition to being sick, crazy and weak. No matter what, he was not going to a psychiatrist. When Mary got home, things would be better. Why was she always out so long?

Although George's behavior suggests a more serious depression, he is resisting getting help, because he fears being seen as mentally sick and fears being stigmatized. He also does not want to upset his family. Unfortunately in our culture, the myths, stereotypes, ideals, and heroes tend to teach us to believe that feelings of sadness, grief, and anxiety are a sign of weakness, are unmanly, and imply self-pity. At the same time, society casts out, withdraws from, and labels as different, ugly, or diseased, those members of society who do not enjoy perfect health.

"Pull yourself up by your bootstraps" is the philosophical advice that has been translated to mean, do not feel or talk about the sadness or any other feeling this problem has caused you. The paradox is that to cope effectively with losses and pain, most people need to express their grief and sadness. Only then can they get to the point where they can pull themselves up by their bootstraps. Allowed to express anger, fear, sadness, and anxiety about the future, loss of roles, friends, and work, most people will then be able to look ahead to the future with increased hope and high expectations for a life worth living. Despite fears about being seen as weak or crazy, it is very important to get medication, psychotherapy, or both when depression has become so severe that the person is unable to function either socially, vocationally, or both.

Family members are also in danger of experiencing depression that escalates beyond the grieving response. It is important for family members to talk about their own feelings of anxiety, anger, and sadness separately and not with the ill or disabled person. Family members sometimes feel very depressed, because they did not believe the ill or disabled person when he was complaining or depressed, and got angry with him or became irritable with him. This guilt (which really is an example of human beings' belief that they can be omniscient and know the unknowable), can precipitate a serious depression. Just like the afflicted person, family members mourn the losses in their lives caused by the illness or disabilities. Usually this mourning does not cause a debilitating depression.

Another important point to remember is not to think that there is a single correct way to feel or react to a given situation. There is no one, right way to feel or react to catastrophic loss. Different people respond differently to life events. Each of us has our own unique ways of understanding what happens to us in life. Some people do not even respond with sadness and grief. The adage "when things get tough, the tough get going" is an example of a more stoic approach to major stresses and changes. Religion and the feeling that sad events in one's life are part of God's plan or are God's will, also serve to reduce the stress of these major life events. Sometimes denial works effectively.

◆ Mary, who had lost both her legs in a serious car accident, could not wait to go to physical therapy. She went twice each day and was now going to speak to her physical therapist about going three times a day. These people really understood her. They knew she was in pain, but they encouraged her to keep going. She would walk again. She knew if she kept going and worked hard, she would be able to put on the prosthesis and walk. She did not believe her physician for one moment. She would show him that he was wrong. After all, it was her body.

Mary believes she will walk again, and her belief helps get her out of bed in the morning and gives purpose to each day. Maybe a day will come when she will have to face the reality of her injury. She will feel the sadness and need to grieve what she has lost, but when that time comes, she may also have shown herself how independent she can be. So sometimes denial is very useful and necessary. It certainly ought not to be tampered with by well-meaning health professionals, or by family when the denial is not getting in the way of progress toward emotional and physical healing. Whatever sadness a person feels, whatever grief he feels, and whenever he feels it in response to his illness, physical disability, or both, it is appropriate and important. But the timing is an individual matter.

At certain times during the year, people are more vulnerable to experiencing renewed feelings of sadness and grief, or depression. These times include anniversaries of the day of accidents, diagnoses, operations, or heart attacks. Holidays often are difficult times of the year, especially when families spent time together or took special trips so they could participate in events together, and are now no longer able to. If it is impossible to attend routine family events or participate in these events in the way one usually did—e.g., dancing at a wedding—the vulnerability is greater. Unfortunately, whenever one can compare a present situation to a former and similar time, the loss is recognized, and feelings of sadness can reoccur.

It is helpful to be aware of occasions and times of the year that hold special significance. If the family anticipates that a day or time of year will be difficult, they can plan to do something that will be distracting or pleasurable that day. It is important that the whole family (or the members who usually participate) be involved in these new plans so that whatever is decided upon is a mutually agreed upon fun event. To sit at home recalling the past and feeling that the future can never be as good, simply increases one's depression and delays the time when one can cope with his altered future and get on with life.

If during these special days, the sad feelings or grief surface, it is important to know that the feelings will pass and that there was a particular reason for their reoccurrence or occurrence. Keep in mind that events which precipitate feelings of grief, sadness, loss of appetite, etc., for a given person, may not be recognized as precipitating events by health-care workers or the family. When a person experiences renewed feelings like this, he may have to search his own mind to find a precipitating factor, but usually there is a plausible reason.

Another thing that can happen is that health professionals and others may misinterpret normal grief reactions as something else. This can happen as early as the first hospitalization or first diagnosis. In the hospital after a spinal-cord injury, mastectomy, chemotherapy, or stroke, for example, patients may feel sad, cry, lose their appetite, feel anxious, sleepless, and in general, fit a picture of depression. These feelings can be misinterpreted, and a nurse or physician may feel that the person needs anti-depressant medication to relieve depression; however, the person is experiencing a normal grief reaction.

Sometimes health-care professionals get scared and think the person is having a mental problem. It is as important for them as for the person suffering the illness, to differentiate between the response to a serious illness or life-altering accident, and a major affective (depressive) disorder. Lying in bed with tubes in your nose, unable to move, scared beyond belief, and uninformed about or unable to understand what is happening, taking medications that might have all sorts of untoward effects, knowing no one, unable at times to talk, lying in an uncomfortable position, feeling all alone and uncertain about your future are sufficient reasons for people to become seriously depressed. Certainly we can expect to experience many symptoms similar to severe depression.

The next few paragraphs describe precipitating situations in which one would expect many people to experience feelings of grief, sadness, or even mild depression as a reaction to the situation.

There are times in rehabilitation for strokes, amputations, arthritis, or other disabilities, when things just do not go well, or rather than improving at a steady rate the person plateaus or even slips back a bit. This is discouraging and may make a person feel inadequate to the task of living and the demands he now has to deal with. It is at those times that he may look like he is depressed and unable to cope but he may be reacting to the moment and the events of the moment. Emotions of rage or grief are not uncommon in this setting either.

The first time a stroke victim, paralyzed on one side and now unable to walk without a wheelchair, gets out of bed, he can develop a series of new complaints like headaches, tiredness, crying, and behavior that appears resistant to his overall recovery. Actually what is happening is that he is for the first time confronting the reality of the changes and the reality of the consequences of the stroke. While in bed, the person appears relatively normal and not paralyzed, and does not have to feel or think about the truth. Once in that chair, it is not easy to deny what has happened. It is also very hard to find himself in a wheelchair and experience his unresponding limbs, with all the attendant and sometimes overwhelming feelings of rage and grief.

The realization of loss of coordination for whatever reason—quadriplegia, multiple sclerosis, cerebral palsy, head injury, stroke, Alzheimer's Disease, Parkinson's Disease, other neurologic diseases, etc., can precipitate sad feelings and certain symptoms because of the loss of dignity involved. The frustration of trying to eat and seeing others try to eat can precipitate loss of appetite and withdrawal.

Recognizing the sexual changes and dysfunction due either to paralysis, loss of functioning, or required medication can also lead to feelings of hopelessness.

The first visit home after a hospitalization for a serious illness that now requires life-style changes or disability, is often an emotional time. Arriving at home to find that you cannot climb the stairs or that your spouse has to help you walk into the house and hang up your coat can bring monumental feelings of grief. Whenever grief and anger reappear or appear, you should ask yourself: "What is happening now that I may be reacting to?" This will help you to understand and to cope.

Sometimes the symptoms of depression will occur as physical symptoms, causing the sufferer to go to his doctor complaining about the physical problems. It is, of course, important to investigate any significant physical symptoms to make sure that some additional organic condition has not arisen. However, if no organic cause can be found for symptoms, it is once again important to ask: "Could there be a precipitating event that would bring back grief and sadness at this time? Why now?" If you think about it, you will nearly always find the reason for the renewed feelings.

Worsening of a progressive disease, reoccurrence of a disease, or a deterioration in a disease that had previously plateaued are all good reasons for new feelings of grief. A reoccurrence after a long period of stability for a multiple sclerosis family, a reoccurrence after many years of cancer, the development of a serious medication side effect when the primary disease has been controlled are examples of these situations. Many times the grief is not recognized for what it is.

What can help relieve or modify these feelings of sadness and discouragement? For some people, it is very helpful to gain information, especially after a diagnosis and during times of discouragement. (See Chapter 1: Learning All about Your Illness.) Gathering and understanding information about their illness helps them to regain a sense of control that the illness has taken away. Reading books and pamphlets about the illness, talking with physicians and other health professionals or others who have the illness helps them gain a feeling of being on top of what is happening to them. If the person is well-educated about his illness, he can make maximal use of diet, exercise, and medication strategies, to help manage the illness or disability, and optimize his medical care.

◆ John had a diagnosis of AIDS. After the initial shock and panic, he began to gain as much information as he could. He talked with his doctor and learned about blood levels, and what was good and what was bad. He learned about the various medications coming from Japan and Europe. He heard one day about a study that was being done at the local university hospital, to test medication to treat AIDS patients who were transfusion dependent, a category, unfortunately, that he had fallen into. He called up the researcher listed in the paper and went for an evaluation. It was a double-blind study, so at first he did not know whether or not he was getting the placebo or the vaccine. However, he had qualified to be in the study, and this gave him a hopefulness he had not felt before. Soon it became clear that he was getting the new medication, as his blood levels improved and he no longer needed transfusions. He was elated. John told his peers at the support groups for AIDS patients he went to, about the medications, combinations of medications, and the study. Through John's efforts, Jim learned about the study, and he qualified as well. John felt a real sense of satisfaction about being able to help someone else qualify for the study.

John's way of coping enabled him to feel in control and on top of his illness. He was actively involved in his treatment. His personal involvement empowered him and took away feelings of helplessness and dependence. He gained personal satisfaction and an increased sense of well being because he could help others as well. The support group members were able to gain from his knowledge. It is important for people who cope by gaining information and becoming involved, to have opportunities to do things, to read, to talk to doctors and professionals who have worked with their illness, and to ask questions and get answers. In this way they become the expert on the topic of their illness or disability. This can help them overcome feelings of sadness and depression.

Adjusting to illness can be greatly facilitated by interacting with others who have faced the same problems. By talking with others, information can be shared, feelings expressed, and the sense of aloneness overcome. An easy way to do this is to join local chapters of national organizations dedicated to research, fund raising, and service to those who have the same illness or disability. These organizations often run support groups or provide home visitors, telephone groups for the home bound, funds for home care, and valuable information and support. Hospitals often have heart clubs, diabetes clubs, and run weekly or monthly meetings for patients and their families who have had coronary artery bypass surgery or strokes. American Cancer Association runs ostomy groups, as well as mixed diagnoses groups.

A patient who had a laryngectomy and lost his voice as a result of surgery, met with several people, some of whom used an electrical device placed on the larynx for speaking and some who had learned esophageal speech. After meeting with them, he felt much less depressed and anxious about this loss and was able to make a decision for himself about which method he wanted to use.

If you are a more private person and groups make you uncomfortable, you can get a name of someone from an association or from a professional whom you can call and set up an appointment to discuss aspects of your illness or disability about which you have questions. This can be done over lunch or at your home. Visiting nurses are another excellent source of information, services, and resources. Visiting nurses' associations provide at-home care, help solve and identify problems, and provide linkage to clergy, physicians, social workers, psychologists, occupational and physical therapists. In addition, they can and often do know of supplies and equipment that can be useful to the home bound.

A key to relieving feelings of sadness, loneliness, and despair is to keep active. The more activities you engage in, the more normal you feel. The more you can restore your life and the things you enjoyed before the illness or disability, the less loss you will feel.

Both family members and the ill or disabled person need to keep expectations high. The worst thing anyone can do to an ill or disabled person is to treat him as an invalid, overprotecting him, and holding him back from doing activities or things for himself. Subtle suggestions that sex or travel are over are usually erroneous and can lead to feelings of sadness and unnecessary feelings of loss. If you have any questions about the advisability of any activity, ask your doctor. Do not automatically eliminate the activity! Do whatever you can do by yourself. Test the limits of your independence. Do not allow others to treat you as an invalid. Get angry about that. Despite subtle suggestions from society that it would be better for you to stay locked away in your room, do not. Find ways to be helpful. Continue working if possible. If not, take over jobs around the house, with the children, and in the community. Find alternatives to whatever you can no longer do, or find alternative ways to do what you used to do. There are opportunities now, even if they are the result of illness or disability, that would not have occurred to you to do before your illness.

Time can be spent with family and children that may never have been possible prior to the illness. Hobbies, languages, gardening, sewing, painting, playing the piano, may now be developed, and may give joy and become a role model for children or other disabled people. Decide what it is that would give you some pleasure, which you never had time to do before, and plan ways to do these things. Even thinking of things you might enjoy that until now you could not do because of time pressures, can relieve feelings of sadness.

Sometimes when one is receiving ongoing treatment for illness, like chemotherapy, it is difficult to feel physically well and hopeful. Often people think about these treatments for days in advance and may even experience symptoms of the chemotherapy before it is given, because of their anxiety and dread. It is true that feelings of sadness and physical discomfort are not just talked away. Recognizing that you have a right to feel awful after chemotherapy is helpful, but try to arrange for something soothing and nice to happen on that day also. A backrub or watching a movie may feel good. Think of what would feel good, talk with family members about what they can do, and plan to do it on that day. Everyone is different, and that is an individual choice. But try to think of something you would enjoy, and plan to do it to take away some of the unpleasantness of the treatment.

The importance of the ill or disabled person maintaining a role in the family, of not lowering expectations for that person, and the importance of finding work and activities in which he/she can be involved, is emphasized throughout the book. If a disability or illness stabilizes, there is more opportunity to resume life activities and work, but if it does not and progressively worsens, then the changes that will be necessary for the future need to be anticipated. By anticipating what will be needed, even if it necessitates a move to a different home, you can prevent chaos and despair when the move is finally essential.

Finally, it should always be remembered that family members who can get together and talk about all these things can help each other cope better. Talking and planning together can lift feelings of hopelessness and feelings of loneliness. Who is involved in these discussions will vary from family to family, and may even include the extended family: brother, sisters, sons, daughters, mothers, fathers, or sometimes just the couple alone.

We feel that it is often useful to include as many people as possible. Family resources can be enormous. Distant relatives can know people, information, and resources of which you were not even aware. Family members besides the immediate family can be called upon for respite support. Vacation homes and vans can be shared. Social support, friends, and family are an important source of comfort, information, and resources. Include friends who want to be a part of your life. Make sure you are not excluding them because of your own sense of shame, or feelings of competition and jealousy. Friends, too, can offer respite help, supplies, vacation ideas, help at home, and loving support.

All this returns a sense of control and order to the ill or disabled person, which are essential feelings for the relief and modification of feelings of grief and despair.

◆ Grief is a response to the losses due to illness and disability. Often it is mistaken for depression.

◆ Get as much information about the illness as you can from physicians, the library, health professionals, and national organizations.

◆ Talk to others with the same problems by joining local chapters of national organizations.

◆ Meet a person with your illness or disability, for lunch or at your home, to ask questions and share experiences.

◆ Keep active.

◆ At certain times of the year and when significant events are about to occur, the ill or disabled person and family members are more vulnerable to experiencing renewed feelings of grief and sadness. Be on the lookout for these times and plan to be with good friends and busy on those days.

◆ Do not allow others to treat you as an invalid.

◆ Get together with the family and talk about all those things that will help you keep active and be helpful. Work together to find alternative ways for you to do what you used to do.

◆ If things don't improve, and sadness, apathy, or thoughts of suicide persist or worsen, get professional help.

CHAPTER 8

Developing New Roles

When illness is serious and debilitating, the traditional roles of breadwinner, nurturer, and chief decision-maker, among others, are often shifted to other members of the family. If this happens by default and without conscious input by the various people involved, the result can be devastating to the ego and dignity of the person who is ill. The extra burden on the other family members can be equally unwelcome. Such role changes reverberate throughout the family and can disrupt its very fabric, as well as its usual social activities and place in the community.

In this chapter, several couples will be used to illustrate some concepts. The first couple, John and Maureen, in which John is stricken in his thirties with multiple sclerosis, will be used to illustrate problems faced by younger families. This family has two school-age children. The second couple, William and Ann, will represent a near retirement-age couple who suddenly have to cope with painful and deforming arthritis. Since some role changes are unique to women, especially when there are still young children, a third set of sketches about Alice and Tim will depict the most common of these. Alice has a progressive hereditary emphysema.

Remember that the illnesses used in the vignettes are purely for illustration; nearly all diseases, if they cause significant fatigue, or physical or mental disability, have the same emotional and social impact.

John and Maureen

◆ John and Maureen had known each other since childhood. They were married in their early twenties and had two children, Kevin, 13, and Susan, 8. As manager of the auto parts division for a major retailer, John had done very well and had a bright future with the company. He was thirty-five when he began to experience episodes of numbness in his right arm that would soon be diagnosed as the first signs of multiple sclerosis.

In the early years of their marriage, Maureen had worked as an elementary school teacher, but she stopped when the children were born. Since John was earning enough to provide a comfortable living, two years ago Maureen had fulfilled her dream of going to work part-time at a boutique, a position that paid very little.

Within six months of his original symptoms, John began to have difficulty with coordination and bladder control and eighteen months later, he was experiencing difficulty walking. He found himself so fatigued many days that it was an effort to get to work. Soon it became clear he could no longer work full-time. In fact, the final blow came one day when his employer called him into the office and suggested he apply for disability.

Disability? At age thirty-seven? Even though he had been ill for almost two years, he wasn't really disabled, was he? How could he tell Maureen? He had very little disability insurance. Who would support them? They had a mortgage on the house; there were ballet and tennis lessons . . .

He went over in his mind at least a hundred explanations of why he was placed on disability, but when he arrived home that night, he couldn't think of anything to tell Maureen. He went to the bedroom and slammed the door!! Maureen had no idea what was happening. John never acted like this. She did not know whether she should try to talk to him or not, so she said nothing.

It can be very frightening and disconcerting to see your spouse in distress. It could be helpful, however, to wait until he comes out before talking to him, though doing so may feel very uncomfortable. John needs some time to prepare himself for the task of telling his wife about a major change in their life. This has been a shock to his ego and self-esteem. Often, although a diagnosis may have been made many months or years ago, it is hard to face the real impact until it affects your job or limits your activities. When there are no major changes in one's life, all that happens is that you say that you have the disease. It is natural and universal to hope that things will change or reverse and return to normal. Now there is a whole other level of adjusting. Now, in this example, John's telling Maureen about losing his job is also admitting he really is sick.

As John prepares himself to break the news, he may be anticipating that Maureen will be angry or will reject him. He may feel like a failure as well as very frightened about his future health and his family's finances. He may feel that all of a sudden at thirty-seven he is looking into a bottomless pit.

If John does not confide in Maureen within a few days, she will need to prod him gently to talk to her. This is a time to make decisions together and not panic. It is normal for them both to feel scared and hurt by their loss and very uncertain about the future. Nevertheless, it is no one's fault that this has happened, and they need each other's support.

After the children have left for school, Maureen can go to John and say, "John, I need to talk with you." She can begin by telling him how worried she feels about him. She can ask him to please let her know what is wrong, encouraging him to think positively and to work with her to solve their problems. In this way she reassures him and lets him know that she will not react negatively. It is very important to keep communication open. In order to do this, one has to first feel free to talk about feelings and concerns without expecting one's spouse, children, or friends to act on them or do anything to make one feel better. Once the person can tell his thoughts and feelings without someone reacting negatively or hysterically, then it is easier to plan constructive solutions together. In other words, a well spouse can be very helpful, if he/she can just listen to the fears and concerns of the ill partner. Let the ill person speak about his concerns without trying to make him feel better by saying for example,"Oh, don't worry about it, that's not going to happen." Nor is it helpful to get overly excited and hysterical, causing the ill person to have to calm you down with

BUILDING A NEW DREAM

words of false reassurances like, "Don't worry, I feel better than I did." This will only cause him/her to feel that speaking to you creates more havoc and tension than already existed. The ill spouse needs encouragement not to feel like a burden, and the spouse or children need to know that they help by doing nothing but listening.

◆ When John was finally able to talk to Maureen about the loss of his job, she confided to him that she had been thinking that she might have to get a full-time job. Maureen thought John would react to this suggestion with great relief, but he looked hurt and said nothing. For several days, John was irritable and criticized everything that she did. He snapped at the children about minor things.

When she was ready to go looking for a job, she asked him to look after Susan when she got home from school. John refused, saying he was not a baby-sitter and had more important things to do.

Not only has John been forced to face the reality of illness, but he has also lost an important role in the family. Although Maureen meant well and thought she was being helpful, she had not included John in making the decision to seek full-time work. Inadvertently, she took another role away from him; that was the role of main decision-maker.

Maureen and John are in this together but are acting separately. John is still struggling with his feelings of guilt and inadequacy since losing his job. How he can now spend his time productively is an important, but as yet, unasked question. John may feel betrayed by his wife. Although John is angry that he is being relegated to baby-sitter and hurt by not being included in the decision about Maureen going to work, he is powerless in this situation, because they really do need her income.

Maureen and John need to find a time when they can be alone. If necessary, children should be sent to visit relatives or friends to allow for this private time. The time should be mutually agreed upon and arranged so that they can talk to each other without interruption about their feelings and fears. A good time for this is often in the evening after dinner.

Not only should John and Maureen talk openly about their disappointments, fears, and resentments, but they can also cry together. Too often one spouse feels that if he/she cries, the partner will feel even worse. Actually, they both often feel better, and they feel as if they are sharing the burden of the illness. Planning together what each person will now be responsible for makes it possible to be supportive of each other. John can get involved with Maureen's job hunting. He was active in hiring personnel in his firm and can coach her on interviewing and writing her resumé. John has skills he may not recognize because he has not needed to use them before. These skills now can be called on so that he can contribute to the new direction the family must go.

Plans for John's time are important too. Spending time with Susan now can give him a chance he might not otherwise have had to become particularly close to her. He will be taking on a nurturing and teaching role his wife is giving up. Maureen can help him learn to nurture and parent their children so that she can continue to be involved in this critical role.

◆ Within two weeks, Maureen was lucky enough to find a teaching job that had been vacated by a pregnant teacher and would pay a much better salary than she was earning at the boutique. Maureen felt some sadness about leaving the boutique but would not let herself think about that. She felt it was selfish to dwell on that when her family needed her and John had this awful illness. She also felt annoyed that she could no longer have time to play tennis with her friends three times a week. She did not mention this to John, because he had so many things on his mind already and this was minor in comparison.

A spouse will feel sad and disappointed about the changes in his/her life-style. Illness strikes at any point in a marriage, and when it does it can cause cataclysmic changes. Current projects like Maureen's boutique may become a luxury and have to be abandoned. Time for leisure activities may now have to be spent at work, doing chores the ill spouse used to do, or caring for the ill person. Often spouses feel that maybe somehow they did something wrong and are being punished. (See Chapter 6: Answering "Why Me?")

Spouses also can feel guilty for feeling angry and disappointed. Anger and disappointment, though, are feelings that are a normal reaction to a life crisis. It is not helpful to discount these feelings by telling yourself that it is silly or bad of you to think this way, but rather they should be recognized and acknowledged. The well spouse has lost things also even if they have their health. They have lost a healthy husband/wife who contributed to the family income and care of the children and provided help around the house. They have to reorganize the way they live their daily lives. Sometimes a spouse considers leaving the marriage. This is also a common reaction and does not mean that one is evil or disloyal. For some marriages, a severe disability or illness does cause so much emotional disruption that divorce is inevitable. If the marriage was filled with conflict before the illness or disability, it may be too hard for a couple to overcome old resentments and find ways to overcome the new difficulties that illness brings in order to feel productive and happy together. However, it is not impossible. Maureen can talk to John about her feelings of loss and disappointment about her job at the boutique and her recreation time. There will be ways for her, with John's cooperation, to arrange time on weekends or after school to play tennis occasionally. If she avoids planning with John new ways to keep up her interests and satisfy these needs, her resentment will grow.

Erroneous feelings that talking about the illness or disability and its impact will upset the sick or disabled person, and make him unhappy or cause a worsening of his disease, prevents open communication. Distance then develops, and couples may begin to avoid each other. A marriage could be endangered at this point, because sometimes a spouse will begin an affair as a way to maintain emotional distance. This is a sure symptom that communication has been closed. When things don't seem to change, professional help can facilitate lines of communication and help focus couples back onto their relationship and ways of being together again. See Chapter 5: Finding and Using Community Resources, for a more detailed discussion about how to find outside help.

◆ Maureen had been working as a teacher for three months. She found she really enjoyed the work, but was also finding it increasingly difficult because she felt like she was holding down two jobs. Not only did she have to do her lesson plans at home in the evening, she also had to make the dinner, do the dishes, do the laundry, arrange car pooling, help with the homework, and make sure all the things around the house stayed in good repair. John, it seemed, spent most of his evening watching TV. If she asked him to help, he was always too tired. In fact, they hardly talked anymore. She was so tired by 10 o'clock, she collapsed in bed.

Beware of this danger. One spouse ends up doing every chore, because the other ill or disabled person cannot or will not. However, John may feel Maureen does not want his help. Maureen may have asked John to do only heavy jobs that he really could not handle. Women have a tendency to feel that they ought to be able to do it all, especially after a couple of requests for help have been turned down. If Maureen were ill, John might consider household help, but this does not even occur to Maureen. There is a real danger that Maureen will become emotionally exhausted. (See Chapter 10: Preventing Emotional Exhaustion.) There is also a real threat to their relationship concealed here. A relationship, under normal circumstances, needs a great deal of time for talking, planning, and accommodating changes in each of the partners. Once illness or disability strikes, these activities are even more vital.

Maureen needs to plan with John to hire household help and to determine which tasks he can do. Then he should be willing to undertake these tasks on a regular basis and not make her nag him to get them done. This way, once the responsibility and work load is shared, the couple will be able to build into their week several hours of time together. Also, though it may take him a while to realize it, John will feel needed and good about having a role in the daily activities of the family.

◆ As John's disease progressed, Maureen found herself doing more and more for her husband. She was helping bathe him, was constantly carrying things to him, specially preparing his food, and managing his medications and doctor's visits. She thought he had become very demanding. He would continually ask for help to do one more thing for him. He seemed to be watching how she did everything, criticizing frequently, and yet every few minutes she heard, "Maureen, get me . . ." She began to ignore his whining and irritating demands. On occasion, she would snap back, "You want me to do everything. I'm doing the best I can."

Maureen felt overwhelmed. She had not gone to a movie or read a book in months. One day in one of her now rare free moments, Maureen remembered a happy time not so long ago when she and John were on a picnic with the children. They had laughed and played together all day. She remembered how they had vowed to do that at least once a year. Now she could hardly envision such an outing. In fact, she could hardly stand looking at him for a whole afternoon. He was not even the same man—just sitting around doing nothing all day. He was not that sick! She wondered how he could stand it and felt a bit ashamed of her own feelings. She felt terrible and as if she wanted to scream. At thirty-seven, her life was no longer fun. How could she live like this?

John has begun to lose control over some basic body functions. He needs help bathing and in cutting up his food. It is a humiliating experience, and he has lost his privacy. He no longer has the physical capacity to be the protector and guardian of his family; his wife has assumed this role. This is a time when an ill or disabled person can become very depressed and feel hopeless about life. However, the well spouse is also under a great deal of stress. He/she can feel overwhelmed by the increased responsibility. Anger may be the normal reaction. "Why does he watch everything I do?"

The disabled person needs to regain some control. By watching how the things he asks for are done, and by finding more things for the spouse to do, he strives to reassert some control over his environment. It is essential that if the ill or disabled member of the family gets very depressed and irritable at this time, and the interpersonal communication breaks down, outside professional counseling be sought. The spouse may also benefit from counseling, especially when he/she begins to feel so angry and overwhelmed that the sick person's demands are ignored. Frequently spouses need to speak to someone about their own misery.

The fact is, Maureen is doing the best she can. This is a hard life for her; it is not what she bargained for. When her workload is particularly heavy, she feels as if she is carrying all the burden, and life seems unfair. Maureen needs to make time for herself. Even though a spouse may be working very hard to keep the family unit afloat, the person often feels guilty that she/he wants some time alone. Feeling guilty because you are well and your spouse is not, can be the feeling behind the sense that you should not take time for yourself. Many times spouses, especially women, think that it is their duty to do everything and not think about themselves. The guilt over thoughts of relaxation is worsened by a disabled spouse who is constantly demanding things, since the implication is that the healthy person, no matter how much they contribute, is not doing enough. While Maureen may acknowledge that she wanted some time, she likely will not plan for it. If she does take it, she may not enjoy herself because of a constant nagging guilt. Particularly when illness causes visible physical changes, the healthy spouse may experience fleeting feelings of repulsion at the body distortions, fleeting feelings of relief that it is not he/she who is suffering the illness, and even occasional feelings of hatred. All these feelings can prevent the healthy person from pursuing personal things, because every time the healthy spouse attempts to do something alone, he/she has an uneasy and troubled feeling that this is being selfish or cruel to the ill person, so it is not done.

Sometimes spouses feel that maybe they did something to cause this terrible thing to have happened. This thought frequently is a way to try to get a feeling of control over the illness. One tries to manage the fear and uncertainty illness brings, by finding a causative agent. Then one might be able to do something about what has happened. It is easier to believe you have caused this, because then you might have the power to undo it. Otherwise, you are helpless and have no control and must rely on others or the unknown. (See Chapter 6: Answering "Why Me?")

Spouses must plan to do the things they have always enjoyed doing. In well-functioning families, whether or not illness is present, couples have to have their time together as well as their time apart. They must pursue their own interests and activities to be fulfilled as individuals. Maureen has to sit down with John alone, or with the help of a counselor, and plan activities they can enjoy together, and other activities they can enjoy apart. To help John regain a sense of control, Maureen can put together a list with him of all the things that need to be done. They can plan when they will get done, and who will do them. John will be in charge of the list, and he will not require that Maureen be his servant. He will be expected to do for himself those things that he is able to do, and if he is not able to do things, he will ask the children as well as Maureen to help him. Some helpful devices can be installed in the home to make him less dependent. For example, if he can no longer dial the telephone, a voice-activated phone can be purchased to allow John to call repairmen or to make business calls without the assistance of family members. All possible equipment that is within the family's means and will allow John to remain independent as long as possible should be bought or rented. Specially designed door knobs or doors that open automatically are often very useful. Giving John responsibility for tasks, even if he is a bit afraid to do them, is also important. It is necessary for both the ill or disabled person and his spouse to overcome the often groundless fears that they will cause more damage by doing various tasks. Family members should have clear guidelines from their doctor about what they can and cannot do. If there are any questions about this, the person's doctor should be consulted so that there are clear expectations for what the ill person and family members can do. Again, more suggestions for the various aids available for disabled persons can be found in Chapter 5: Finding and Using Community Resources and in Appendix 2.

◆ One morning a few months after Maureen started working full-time, she found the basement flooded with water when she went to do the laundry. "Oh, damn it," she said aloud, but without another thought, she picked up the phone and called the plumber. As she finished making arrangements for him to repair the pipes, she realized that she had never done this sort of thing before; her prowess made her feel good. As she was leaving for work, she mentioned to John that the plumber would be coming. "Why didn't you tell me," he retorted. "I would have taken care of it." Feeling hurt and unappreciated, Maureen decided it would be less of a hassle to not even mention problems like this to John in the future.

Having spent so much time learning to be in charge and taking charge, it is natural for Maureen to automatically do what needs to be done. In fact, she feels a sense of pride and accomplishment in being able to handle things on her own. Inadvertently, Maureen forgets to make space for John.

It does not even occur to Maureen to suggest that John take care of the problem. Since she has assumed so much other responsibility, she takes for granted that she must take action in an emergency. When John appears ungrateful, Maureen feels unappreciated. John, on the other hand, is feeling impotent and a burden. His sense of guilt and shame at his inability to protect his family overshadow any sense of pride he might have felt for his wife's accomplishment. Men in our society frequently are burdened with the belief that if they do not do the jobs that are considered men's jobs, such as taking care of emergencies, they are unmanly. These thoughts lead to feelings of guilt and shame, such as John may be feeling. Ultimately, Maureen's self-esteem and position in the family is strengthened, and John's is weakened.

This can be a threat to the basic structure of the family. Maureen may pull back and not inform John about what is happening with the family affairs. This will increase his sense of isolation, dependency, and uselessness. Maureen needs to recognize the growing ease she feels with responsibility. While this is a positive outcome of the assuming of new roles and important in the adaptation of their relationship, John's feelings of being unneeded and dependent cannot be ignored. John can probably handle much of the running of the house, especially with the help of special devices we mentioned above. Certainly, if John can supervise and thus maintain some control of the household, it will free up some of the time Maureen has been wanting. John may even be able to work at home. For this arrangement to succeed, the two of them will have to sit down and divide up the types of responsibilities each has. Then they will have to stick to it. If Maureen steals John's responsibility by automatically calling the repairman, for example, nothing will be accomplished. Maureen, as well as John, can feel a sense of confidence and enjoyment from seeing themselves succeed in their new roles.

◆ One afternoon, Susan, a third grader, brought some of her schoolmates home for peanut butter sandwiches. By the time John, who was napping, realized this, peanut butter covered not only the countertop in the kitchen but wide expanses of the floor as well. Angrily, he ordered Susan and her friends to clean up the mess. "No," she said, "Mommy will do it when she comes home." And then she left the house with her entourage. More and more, John was noticing that Susan and Kevin would mind their mother, but not him, and would ask her permission to do things rather than his. Now he felt she was deliberately disobeying him, because physically he could not stop her. John used to feel so close to Susan, and now he was not sure he even liked her anymore.

Children's reactions to parents' illnesses are often very strong and frequently not verbally expressed. Children, regardless of age, pick up emotional and physical changes in their parents and harbor thoughts and feelings that could be unnecessarily harsh or negative. Children are likely to fear that their parent might die, that they might have caused the problem, or that they too may get ill or disabled. They may feel scared as well as guilty because they find the illness or disability disgusting and do not want to be near their parent. Children express these feelings through their behavior. Sometimes they become exceedingly good. They do everything they are told, even though before the illness they were able to disagree or refuse to do some things. Sometimes children disobey and become very difficult to manage. Susan, in this vignette, might be displaying that kind of response to her father's illness and the changes in her mother's time at home. Changes in behavior at school such as fighting and isolation from peers, and complaints from teachers that homework is not getting done and grades are falling, are warning signs that the child is having reactions to the illness or disability in the family. When this occurs, it is very important and helpful to inform school guidance counselors and teachers about the illness or disability and about the changes that are happening at home. Teachers and counselors can give the children more attention, talk to them about their feelings, and be a resource to the family.

Teenagers may express their feelings and reactions by being truant at school, by failing, by delinquent behavior—stealing, or taking the car without permission—or by drug and alcohol abuse. Because teenagers are very concerned with appearances and their own acceptability with their peers, they may be very embarrassed around their ill or disabled parent. They may not want to invite friends to their home or have parents attend school functions. This may be difficult for the parents while it is going on, but in time teenagers do mature. It is important for the ill or disabled parent not to give up important, once-in-a-lifetime events, such as grad-uations, concerts, sports events, etc., because of their teenagers' insecurities. Firmly, let them know you plan to attend these things, but give them permission to spend time with their friends if they prefer. (See Chapter 15: Meeting Family Social Responsibilities.)

Frank discussions telling children the nature of the illness or disability, the present-day consequences, and the possible future losses can ease many of their fears. Allowing them to express their feelings and concerns about the illness and sharing your feelings with them can be very helpful to them. Younger children need to know only what they have questions about. Take your lead from them. Let them ask questions and respond to what they are fo-cusing on. You may have to be the one to initiate the conversation. "Susan, I notice you have been disobeying me a lot lately, and I don't understand what is making you act that way. Can you tell me what is bothering you?" may be enough to get the conversation going, but you may have to say, "Is it my disease and my paralysis that is bothering you?" This allows most children to open up, once they realize it is alright to talk about the illness and their fears.

If they are not asking about future losses in their parents' func-

BUILDING A NEW DREAM

tioning yet, wait awhile and take it step by step. As new changes occur, discuss it with them. Make sure they know what is happening, and let them talk to you about how they are feeling and what they are thinking. Let them know what you are feeling and thinking as the illness progresses and more changes occur. If you do not forget that they are reacting and are very frightened because they fear the loss of their parent, and find time to talk to them, they can adjust very well. Children like to feel helpful. Find ways they can participate and help the ill or disabled parent.

If very self-defeating behaviors—poor school performance, dropping of activities, etc.—start to occur, it is very important to meet with a professional. A meeting with a family therapist, clergy, or school counselor to help the whole family talk about their feelings and give their reactions to the changes can be exceedingly helpful, no matter what the ages of the children are. A therapist can help open up communication, which may be hard for a family that is not accustomed to sharing these kinds of feelings, or aware that there can be such strong reactions in children. Also, a therapist knows what the feelings might be that children and parents experience, and can be very helpful in educating the family about these matters. Many times parents misunderstand their children's behavior and are very hurt by it, and are angry at them. Therapists can explain to parents what the behavior really is all about and allow the whole family to improve the way they communicate, so that these behaviors no longer occur, or at least are improved.

In addition, especially when there is a disability involved, or when illness seriously affects the parent's ability to be mobile, the couple needs to teach young children to respect the authority of the affected parent. A child must learn he cannot run away from a physically limited parent. It will not be tolerated by either spouse. Parental discipline will be maintained. The well parent needs to confer with her/his spouse before decisions involving the children are made. Rules for the children's behavior should be reviewed and adhered to by both parents. An illness or disability does not take away parenting responsibilities, or the ability to parent. Parenting needs to be a couple-responsibility. Under normal circumstances, couples need to discuss together how they want to respond to their children's behavior. They have to agree about rules and the consequences for breaking the rules, prior to telling their children. Illness or disability does not change the need for parenting to be a couple-responsibility. Unwittingly, the disabled or ill parent does less and is asked to do less. This may be the result of the ill or disabled parent's feeling that he/she can't control the child anymore. This parent may also be less involved, because when an ill or disabled parent is involved, the limitations of the disability or illness must be faced. Figuring out ways to keep the ill or disabled parent involved and in charge is the challenge for both parents. Again this challenge is best met if the parents discuss what they see is happening with their child and make a joint decision about what they want to do about it, and which one of them will do it. Each time a situation arises, the parents have to have this conversation. When children see that their parents agree and that they back each other up, they do not try to pit one against the other. The able-bodied or well spouse can be more attuned to the ill or disabled parent's withdrawal from active control of their children. When a spouse sees this, it is a time to flag it. "Flagging" disturbing behavior of a spouse, child, lover, family member, or friend for later discussion, is a useful technique. Maureen can say to John, "John, I am flagging your behavior. You did not stop Susan from running around the A&P today. You left that to me when I know you can handle that. Let's sit down later and talk about it. O.K.?"

◆ John had made extensive preparations for a week's vacation to a cousin's farm in Oregon when Maureen and the children had time off. John really looked forward to spending time with his son, now a teenager, and he was going to teach Kevin and Susan something his own father had taught him—how to harvest honey from the beehives on the farm. That time with his father on their own farm was one of John's fondest childhood memories. He knew he no longer had the physical strength to remove the honeycombs, so he made arrangements with a farmhand to accompany him and the children to the hives. He explained to Kevin how to protect himself from the bees, and told him how Kevin's grandfather had started the honey business in that part of the state and had developed ways to place the hives so the bees would make the most honey.

John watched while the farmhand guided Kevin through the process of gathering the honey. Kevin was pleased and excited and did not get stung once. Susan could hardly wait to tell her mom. John watched his son and tried to remember the same moments with his father. To his surprise, he felt an emptiness and disappointment and none of the satisfaction he had expected; it seemed completely different from when he did this with his own father.

John has accomplished something important. He has organized and put together a vacation and an activity that he can share with his wife and children. The vacation gives Maureen a well-earned break as well. By setting up a mutual activity, he is also helping to strengthen the family unit.

But it seems that John is devaluing his role as organizer and prime mover, because he can't handle the hives. He feels empty and disappointed, because it hurt to have to rely on someone else, and it certainly was a reminder that his illness was progressing.

Kevin and Susan, however, were delighted. Children need to know that their parents care enough about them to put energy and time into arranging an activity just for all of them. If a parent is disabled or ill, they fear that these activities will never occur again. It is John, not his children, who is suffering from the inability to gather the honey. This feeling is a feeling of loss that an ill or disabled person often experiences as he/she does take part again in activities they used to do before becoming ill or disabled. It is at these times that changes in functioning are most apparent to the ill or disabled. In time the focus of enjoyment needs to shift from doing the activity itself to the experience of making it happen and sharing it with one's children. Sometimes parents worry that if they cannot do the activities with their children, then they are depriving them of a role model. This is a normal reaction during illness because we tend to think of ourselves as models for our children in terms of physical things we can do. Physical activities are important to both men and their sons, and women and their daughters. Parents believe that if they throw a ball or fish or ski, then their child learns to do these activities. Children can learn activities, however, by being exposed to them, and not necessarily only by watching their parents doing them. Parents can teach by talking their children through tasks. Parents can be just as effective at role modeling by creating the opportunities for the child. An ill or physically disabled person has usually not lost the ability to create these opportunities, and it is not only his right, but his responsibility to his children, to see that they have these opportunities.

John will have periods of sadness about his own physical losses. He is grieving. Although his adaptation is good and he was able to plan this vacation, he is not able to feel good about this accomplishment yet. He is still very aware of what is gone. It is like mourning for a lost friend or relative. Every once in a while, one is reminded that they are no longer around, and one feels the sadness. In time, this will happen less often, and John will be able to focus on the time spent with his children and wife and derive pleasure from it that is untainted by the sadness of his losses. If not, he should seek outside assistance.

William and Ann

◆ William and Ann had been married for thirty-five years when William developed rheumatoid arthritis in his hands and knees. Since he was a graphic artist, the arthritis made it particularly difficult for him to do his work. While this couple had been through many minor problems and illnesses during their long marriage, nothing had threatened their life-style and well being like this illness. They had two children, Michael, thirty-four, and Peter, thirty, and five grandchildren ranging in age from four to fourteen.

Soon it became apparent that William would have to consider an early retirement because of his physical disability, and because the pain and fatigue accompanying his illness made even small problems at work seem overwhelming. Yet, at fifty-seven, William felt too young to retire. Ann, herself, had diet-controlled diabetes and angina pectoris, and had to be conscious of her own diet and health.

Ann felt very frightened and worried. If William retired, how would they survive? They had already used much of their savings to put Peter through college and graduate school, and had just recently built up another nest egg.

William was relieved that he had already put his children through college, but he felt worried that there would not be enough money for their retirement years, and they would have to live at a lower standard of living. He found it difficult to think about the money situation and spent a great deal of time looking for a cure for his arthritis.

Ann, on the other hand, thought about the potential financial difficulties nearly every day and found that whenever she mentioned it to William, he either left the room or complained about the pain in his hands.

Soon they found they were hardly talking to one another, and when they did, they yelled.

For some older couples, there are great fears about poverty in retirement, the supposedly golden years. When such anxiety occurs, it is very hard to focus one's thoughts on the cause of the anxiety. It is much easier to cope by distancing oneself from the problem. William does this by thinking only about curing his arthritis which, if that were possible, would remove the fear of losing his income, and restore his life to normal. There is a possibility that William will spend much time and money consulting many physicians vainly in search of a cure, rather than assessing and investigating his potential financial resources.

Ann takes a different approach to adversity. Her way of coping with problems is to worry. There are a number of things to worry about. Not only is she also frightened about poverty in her old age, but she may also be fearful William will die and leave her to fend for herself. The worry here is about how she will survive if that should happen. Ann also is aware that she has health problems, and watching William deteriorate could make her keenly aware that she may get sicker.

Her way of confronting problems puts pressure on William. Not only does she ask him to listen to her fears, but she also wants him to do something. This makes him feel helpless. What can he do? Since William is coping by ignoring the problems for now, communication is becoming very difficult. William's and Ann's styles of coping are so different that it puts them in conflict with one another. The fighting and silences are a symptom that they are not effectively resolving their concerns and problems. They are now afraid of insulting each other, and the breakdown of communication is compounded. At the moment, they each feel isolated in their own way from one another. When fears begin to get unmanageable, it is more important than ever to be able to problem solve. By coming up with a variety of possible plans to combat the problems, fears are reduced. Problem solving, which results in several contingency plans, restores a sense of control to the family.

At this moment, either William or Ann has to remind the other that they have stopped talking. Since they have lived together for a long time, it is very likely that one or the other will make this move. Once they have flagged that they are angry and silent, they can plan a time to talk. Sitting down together after lunch, Ann or William can suggest that they need to plan and figure out exactly what their financial situation is. If this is usually William's job, then Ann can suggest that he check into it. This might be a good time to bring in the family accountant, lawyer, or a close relative to sit down with William and Ann to go over their financial resources and explore alternatives. Far too often, older couples do not know what their resources or choices are. They may have no idea how much money they need to live on, whether or not insurance policies have disability clauses, or whether they may be eligible for disability pensions. One way to reduce financial fears is to know exactly what a family's assets are, and to formulate a plan of action for the future based on that information. (For more discussion of this sort of problem, see Chapter 14: Handling Changes at Work.) When they have a better idea of their financial situation, William and Ann will be calmer; and then they may be able to talk more easily about how they were feeling, and why they were so upset.

◆ For years Ann had looked forward to the time they would spend together after William's retirement. But things were not turning out as planned. She had envisioned them going out for walks together and enjoying each other's company. She knew William had pain, but she often thought he was exaggerating. In any case, her patience was running thin. Sometimes she almost accused him of faking but always stopped herself in time. She was tired of being awakened every night to rub his aching legs, or fetch his painkillers. With her diabetes and angina, she needed plenty of sleep herself: He seemed to have forgotten all about her health. Maybe, she thought to herself, she really did not like having him around that much anymore. She had to do all the yard work and many other things that she had come to depend on him to do. Now she had to open her own jars, change all the light bulbs, and carry the groceries. She began to feel angrier and angrier each day, yet she was ashamed of herself for feeling this way.

The quality of Ann and William's life has deteriorated, and the demands of the illness have become burdensome. Ann had not anticipated being tied down like this. She is unable to get her needs met, she feels she has to respond to her ill husband, and she has to take on more chores at a time when she had expected fewer. Who is doing things for her? It is annoying to be awakened each night. One expects this from a child but not from one's husband. Her anger and resentment at this intrusion, though, makes her feel guilty; he is her husband and he is in pain.

Ann's unhappiness has a lot to do with her disappointment, for these are hardly the fun-filled retirement years. If they are going to be able to make these years as pleasurable as possible, it is going to be necessary for them to begin talking about what they each need, and to begin finding some solutions. Ann will feel far less angry when some appreciation of her needs is demonstrated. She needs to feel like a wife and partner, not a servant. Ann may end up feeling like a servant, because she may believe that a good wife should do all these things for her husband, especially if he is sick. And because of these beliefs, it may be very hard for her to stop doing everything for him even though she feels like a servant.

This is not realistic. If she continues to try to do all these things, she will continue to feel resentful and angry. It is necessary for her to learn that she can still be a good wife and not do all these things. She and William need to talk about Ann's feelings. William needs to take on more of the responsibility for his own care. For example, Ann needs help around the house. It is important that she be relieved of some of the daytime chores. A homemaker or housekeeper can be hired to come in once or twice a week to help Ann. Also it might help to call a visiting nurse to evaluate the situation and recommend outside resources. The visiting nurse can also make suggestions about how things can be done differently in the home.

In the evening, William's painkillers and a glass of water should be placed by his bed when he is ready to go to sleep. He should be encouraged not to awaken Ann to rub his legs; Ann's sleep should be as much a priority to him as it is to Ann, since her health is at stake too. This need of William's can be controlled in some other way. Perhaps he can rub his own legs, purchase an electric massager to use, try a heating pad, or get up and walk around when he has cramps at night.

◆ William and Ann had enjoyed playing golf together for years. In fact, Ann had never played without William. However, recently she had been doing many things alone for the first time. So when her friend Aggie called and invited her to play nine holes, she felt excited and said she would ask William if he minded. When she asked him, William began complaining about all the things he could not do anymore, and ignored her question. Ann decided he was ignoring her and decided to go golfing anyway. She did not have much fun, though, because she had a nagging sense of guilt about leaving William alone. This was the first time in thirty-five years that she had gone against his wishes.

Illness changes the marital relationship. The healthier person wants to continue doing on his or her own, some of the same things that were done as a couple before. These activities are still enjoyable to the unaffected spouse. The ill or disabled person has to give up his role as a companion, a loss which is often hard to face. It is common to have a feeling that life—and the spouse—is leaving him behind. Instead of discussing these feelings of loss, concerns about becoming a burden, and fears of the future, the ill person often responds with criticism and complaints. The well spouse has to go on with his/her life and finds it unpleasant to be around a complaining person all the time. As a result, the real feelings underlying the complaining go unexpressed, and a chasm develops in the relationship.

It is important for the well spouse to continue the activities he/she finds enjoyable, and it is as important for the ill or disabled spouse not to make the well person feel guilty in doing so.

One thing a couple can do is sit down together and plan activities the couple can do together, and exactly when they are going to do them. These might include going to movies, visiting friends, or other things they have enjoyed together over the years. They also should plan solo activities that William can enjoy while Ann is out playing golf. The well spouse can openly acknowledge that he/she will be going out to do something they formerly did together, and that the partner's participation is missed.

If there are organized times and events that are still shared, it makes things feel less hopeless and lonely. Someone can visit with William, or he can pursue his own interests while Ann is out. William can also use this time to get to know his grandchildren better, or to visit with his sons. An open environment for discussion and planning will allow both William and Ann to satisfy their needs, even though they need to make some changes in their former life-style.

◆ Ann found herself calling her eldest son, Michael, more and more to help her fix things around the house, like changing the storm windows to screens, trimming the shrubbery, and sealing the driveway. She had never learned to drive, and she needed someone to take her to the grocery store after William's fingers became too weak to hold the steering wheel, let alone carry the groceries. William was relieved that Michael was available to help his mother, but at the same time, felt himself to be a burden and found himself snapping at Michael when he did not even mean to.

Oldest children often are called upon to help when parents become ill. Though the parents may be grateful, it highlights what they can no longer do. William is forced to recognize his growing limitations as head of the house, with each additional responsibility his son assumes. The feeling of becoming a burden is really an expression of despair over the loss of independence. At the same time, there is a sense of relief at being taken care of and not having to do so many things as before, or worry about how they will get done.

Michael's presence is a reminder of the loss of youth and the continued loss of usefulness. There is a normal wish to be young and strong again. A feeling of inadequacy at Michael's strength and ability to take care of Ann is also a normal reaction of a father in William's position. Snapping at Michael is one way to express these feelings of jealousy and despair, though William's feelings may be subconscious, and he may not realize why he is reacting this way to his son's helpfulness. If a father finds he is reacting this way toward his sons, or a mother who is ill toward her daughters, he or she might examine whether some of these feelings are below the surface.

The ill or disabled spouse will find it helpful to ask the son or daughter to sit down and talk. This can be a time to reminisce, or talk about the child's family concerns, and future hopes and plans. It may be a time to offer some advice. Providing the child with a listening ear and some family history can make the parent feel important, and re-establish the father-son or parent-child relationship. The parent will feel less of a loss of his role as caretaker for the family. A child concerned about the ill parent can seek him/her out to ask advice on parenting or being a good spouse, or to just talk about the past and future. This is a new role for the ill or disabled parent, which replaces the lost role and reduces the jealousy and anger.

In fact, it may be a chance to pass on family lore, an opportunity often lost, because the family members never seem to get around to talking about it. Finding new roles brings comfort and closeness at a time when the ill or disabled person is most in need of these things. This is much harder to do if feelings of sadness, anger, and guilt have not been stated openly. Just being able to state these feelings often makes a person feel much better. The person with these feelings needs to be allowed to state them without negative responses or hurt feelings on the part of the other person; similarly, the person stating his feelings ought not to demand that the other person do something about them. How could they be changed anyway?

In order to be able to express their feelings openly, the family members must realize that what keeps them from talking is often fear of hurting the feelings of the ill or disabled person. Not to express these sentiments, however, is likely to result in much greater distress in the family. If families have never been able to speak openly about their feelings, it might help to meet with a professional for just that purpose. A pastoral counselor, a social worker, or a psychologist can help the family openly discuss their feelings and learn how to do this in an ongoing, nonhurtful way. Sometimes just knowing that it won't hurt the ill or disabled person to hear how family members feel, makes it easier to try to have such a conversation. When talking to a family member about your feelings, always begin with "I think" or "I feel." Remind the person to whom you are speaking that they do not have to do anything but listen to you. You don't want them to make you feel better or to be different. You just want them to listen to you. You can also say that you don't want to hurt their feelings, and you hope that you won't; but you want to find a way to talk with them so you can be helpful to them and to yourself. Talking to a family member, without blaming them or accusing them of doing wrong and mean things, allows them to listen to what you are saying, and then to possibly decide to try to be different. You cannot have a conversation if each person can only accuse and blame the other.

◆ As William's arthritis caused more physical disability, he had to make more frequent visits to the doctor. He had to call Michael more and more to drive him. Michael's wife, Judy, felt growing resentment. She felt Michael was missing too much work and neglecting his own family because of his sense of responsibility toward his father. She suggested Michael ask his brother, Peter, to do some of the chauffeuring. When Michael did not get around to doing this, Judy called Peter's wife and suggested that they assume some of the responsibility for William and Ann. Peter interpreted this as an insult, and soon the two brothers were hardly speaking to each other.

The time during which a family member is slowly worsening, is a very stressful period for the whole family. Watching one's sibling or parent deteriorate over months or years is emotionally and physically draining. It is difficult to balance responsibilities to one's parents and one's responsibilities to wife and children. One way to handle the intensity and anxiety, and avoid exhaustion trying to please everyone, is to distance oneself from the problem and from other relatives, like siblings. The result can be that one sibling is doing all the work. When this happens, family feuding is common. Judy's anxiety is about her husband's health and well being, and the well being of her own family. She sees his growing involvement with his father as threatening their own family relationships. She is concerned that Michael will become exhausted and something will happen to his health.

It is important that responsibility for the ill or disabled parent be shared by the children, but Judy's calling her sister-in-law to suggest this has only created more bad feelings and anger. A joint family meeting or Sunday get-together to discuss the problem is a far more open and cooperative approach. Michael needs to initiate this. Michael may have hesitated to ask Peter for help because of his strong sense of responsibility. It is not uncommon for eldest children to take on all the responsibility for the family. In many families one child, usually the eldest, takes on most of the responsibility and forgets to delegate; meanwhile, younger children become used to the idea that their elder brother or sister is taking care of things. They frequently will say that there is not anything they can do, because attempts on their part to help are usually turned down by the eldest son or daughter. After a while, younger children do not even try anymore. Therefore, Michael not only has to delegate, but he has to let Peter help. Peter, on the other hand, has to insist that there be a role for him helping his parents.

One way to do this is to delegate specific jobs to everyone. The two families can create a specific plan at a family meeting. They can talk weekly over the telephone to review how things are working out. As their father's or mother's condition changes, they can rework the plan. Their father is not always going to be stable, and division of responsibilities needs to be written down or talked about as part of an ongoing evaluation of the situation. Once an

BUILDING A NEW DREAM

agreement for division of responsibility is worked out, the two families have to stick to it. Each should set aside special times to spend with his spouse and children too, so they are not neglected.

Peter, Michael, and their wives need to make these practical plans as well as talk about their reactions to their father's losses, the changes in him, and his eventual death. The two brothers need to actively work on re-establishing their relationship now. This includes concerns they each may have about who will be responsible for their mother financially and physically—or for their father should their mother die first.

Sometimes, when one child must take on most of the responsibility, he may have trouble coping with the new demands and may need to speak with a professional counselor. This is a time when physical symptoms such as headaches, pain, ulcers, and diarrhea may occur. Having physical symptoms might be a clue that something emotional is going on for this child. Again, if all the members of the family are asked to share the responsibilities resulting from the illness or disability, and they have a constant ongoing communication to check on things, family feuds and symptoms of illness in the caretakers can be prevented.

◆ William not only enjoyed golf with his wife but had a weekly tennis date with either Michael or Peter. He was very proud of being able to keep up with his sons, and that they wanted to play with him. It also helped them maintain close relationships, because they used these opportunities to confide in one another. When William could no longer do physical things like this, his family noticed that he was becoming more and more reclusive and introverted. It was difficult to draw him into a conversation, and he did not even want to go out for drives.

The loss of this important part of his relationship with his sons, and the loss of his role as a virile and functioning man in his fifties who could keep up with his much younger sons, is a double blow to William's ego and self-esteem. His response is to withdraw emotionally and become very depressed. Although it may be difficult to speak openly about his disappointments, fears, anger, and sense of uselessness, it is important and could allow him to find new ways to relate to his sons. If this is hard for a spouse to do alone, then one or two meetings together with a professional counselor or family therapist may be very helpful. Self-help groups—available through organizations of persons with similar disease or local hospitals or mental-health associations—of families facing similar problems are sometimes available to help in sorting out these feelings. Also, it may be easier for a person to talk about these things with a sibling or a close friend than it is for him to talk with more directly involved family members.

There is nothing mentally wrong with William. He is feeling what a person normally feels at such a time. The problem is that withdrawing, losing hope, and losing close relationships is the result of not being able to express these feelings openly with at least one other person. This leads to further isolation and depression.

◆ One of the biggest joys in Ann's and William's life had been the birth of their first grandchild. They had looked forward to doing all the things that doting grandparents do with their grandchildren. William had vowed to spend the time with his grandsons that he had been unable to spend with his own sons. He would teach them to golf and play tennis. He might even travel with them. Now he rarely wanted them around. He felt tired all the time, and their playful roughhousing caused him a lot of pain. He often yelled at them and noticed that they hardly ever came to the house anymore.

Two losses are occurring here. William has lost whatever enjoyment he could have had by being with his grandchildren, and they have lost an important role model and mentor. The family has also lost the extra time and help that grandparents offer when they take the children. None of this is really necessary as long as William's own children recognize the importance of keeping this relationship functioning. The grandchildren and William can still do things together. They have to prevent family communication from breaking down. One way to do that is to find alternative ways for William to be with his grandchildren. The children really love being together and talking together. That is what is really important, not the specific activities that are undertaken.

William is mourning his losses indirectly through his withdrawing from his grandchildren. Seeing their energy and health, while gratifying to him, also are a reminder of his losses. Feeling helpless and useless because he cannot do things, he devalues what he still can do. He also does not realize that he can take his mind off his own problems if he begins planning activities with his grandchildren. If he actively seeks their companionship, they will respond to him. William can read to them, tell them stories, pass on family lore, play games with them, listen to music with them, listen to their problems, and offer them advice.

Grandchildren may begin to have problems in school, or think about and speak about dying. These symptoms may reflect their concerns about tension in the family and the illness of their grandparent, as well as their fears of death and illness. Grandchildren can react very strongly because of their special attachment to their grandparents. However, their emotional response often gets overlooked. They may have fears and issues that need expressing too. Often grandchildren get isolated from grandparents and do not see them as much, because the parents keep them apart as a way of protecting the grandchildren from sad feelings or fear. There may also be unfounded feelings that the grandparent's health will be harmed. However, the way for children to handle fears and anxiety is to see their grandparents and have opportunities to ask questions and talk about their feelings.

Talking to the grandchildren about their lives and how they feel about the grandparent's illness is often very important to children, and parents frequently do not take the time to do this. Grandparents also seem to have more patience, especially with older children. The grandchildren often have special memories of their grandparents and cherish these moments all their lives.

Unfortunately, what may happen when a grandparent has a serious illness or disability, is that they miss these really unique and satisfying opportunities. Instead they focus on their illness and losses, as if somehow that would make the illness disappear. Irritable and complaining, the grandparent finds himself isolated and lonely when he could have easily avoided that by recognizing the treasures that could have been shared with the grandchildren. The grandparent may well have to make the first move in re-establishing the relationship, but the rewards will be well worth the effort.

Alice and Tim

◆ Alice, forty-two, had been battling hereditary emphysema for twenty years. Recently, Alice found herself so short of breath that she could only walk about ten feet without having to stop and catch her breath. Not only was this very frightening, but it also made it impossible to do many of the household tasks she had to do. Tim, Alice's forty-eight-year-old husband, ran a small business and could not help with the housework or with the care of their four children, Penny, sixteen; John, twelve; Nancy, eight; and Jill, four. As a result, Alice found herself turning to Penny for more and more help. Penny had to go shopping, bring in the groceries, cook the meals, and get Nancy and Jill ready and into bed. Alice thought now and then about how awful it would be without Penny and hoped that Penny meant it when she said she did not mind helping. Alice wanted to believe that Penny really did not mind, but lately Penny was staying out very late; and last Saturday night, she had come home drunk.

Adolescence is the time when families experience the stress of a child's effort to separate and begin developing an identity, and to begin acting on his/her own values. It is a time when teenagers rebel and focus outside the family. Penny is unable to take these important steps, because she is being asked to act as a parent with the responsibilities of caring for her brothers and sisters. Penny's family must be careful not to expect too much from her. Her natural development can be interfered with, and she may not learn how to form relationships (which are necessary for her to grow up) outside her family.

Many children in this position do not leave home for years after most of their peers have left to establish their own households. After the death of the parent, they may remain to care for the younger children and father. Penny shows signs of experiencing the stress of the responsibility placed on her. Though she may not realize it, her drinking and staying out late are her ways of expressing her frustration about the demands that have been placed on her. She probably feels she cannot tell her mother, who is so ill and who may die, that she would rather spend more time with her own friends. It is normal for the maturing teenager to need to spend more time away from the home. Normal anger toward parents and fantasies of one's own lover or husband and children may be suppressed in the face of the overwhelming responsibilities of a parent's severe illness. The adolescent may feel guilty for wanting to strike out on her own. She may consider it disloyal and threatening to the family to even think about her own needs in the face of a parent's severe illness. This guilt may be reinforced by well-meaning relatives or a parent who feels that taking on the ill person's responsibilities is the teenager's duty. The family can become dependent on the adolescent; it is tempting to push the teenager into the role of "mother" or "father" because it minimizes the family disruption and allows most members' lives to continue without much change.

An adolescent should be allowed to develop in as normal a way as possible. It is not the adolescent's responsibility to be mother or father. Tim needs to be more involved in decisions with Alice about who will help her. All the children should share the chores. Organizations like the local American Lung Association or visiting nurses can be called to make suggestions about support services for the family. Household help and baby-sitters can be hired; sometimes relatives will help. The working father may need to rearrange his work schedule. All the children's needs, including Penny's, must be considered. She certainly may be able to take on some increased responsibility, but she must be allowed time for her own activities.

The amount of parenting of the younger children expected of Penny should be carefully thought out and discussed with Penny, and once decided, the limits adhered to.

◆ Recently, as Alice's breathing had worsened, she had been sleeping a great deal. She spent long periods of time now alone in her room. More and more she was sending the girls, Nancy and Jill, over to her sister's house. Alice's younger sister, Helen, lived only a few blocks away. Helen was noticing a change in Jill and

Nancy. Both girls seemed to need a lot of attention. They would hang onto Helen and want to be held and kissed. Jill was sucking her thumb often, a habit she had stopped a year earlier. Nancy kept wanting to hold Helen's hand. Helen found herself giving a lot of time and affection to the girls but also found herself worrying about the future demands on her, though she felt she would do anything for her sister.

Serious illness has a devastating effect whenever it strikes, but when children are young and need mothering, it is especially devastating and untimely. Jill and Nancy are missing the nurturing their mother provided before she became so ill that she needed all her energy to cope with her illness. Not only does Alice's illness prevent her from being able to give her daughters the love and attention they need, she is also deprived of the enjoyment of watching them grow and of sharing experiences with them. They, in turn, are deprived of the attention, love, and role model a mother usually provides. Children's reactions to the seriousness of their parent's illness may vary, but to feel secure they need to maintain a close relationship with the well parent. They need to be assured that someone is still available for them and will not leave them.

Unfortunately, the working spouse experiences increasing stress as well in these circumstances. It becomes tempting to increase the time spent at work as a way of avoiding the stresses within the family. Yet, Tim's children desperately need his emotional support, and he needs theirs. It is a time when he must take on a part of Alice's role, which will provide continuity and cohesiveness. Alice's loss of her mothering role and inability to care for the needs of her children is depressing and difficult for her. She must be careful not to withdraw and become emotionally separated from her youngest children. Other family members like Helen are helpful, but their generosity should not be abused, because they may become overburdened and resentful.

Alice and her children need time together. Alice can still show her children affection and attention, if it is planned and arranged in a quiet place where there are no outside distractions and she does not have to be active. They can read together, watch television together, play board games, work on hobbies, etc. If Alice can be transported in a wheelchair or motorized chair, they might go to the park or on short walks. The whole family can participate in planning these kinds of activities. Tim can talk with his daughters, and they can come up with some ways the girls can be with their mother. That way he participates also.

If the ill or disabled parent has become isolated and remains disinterested in making plans for time together with the children, then it may be necessary to get professional help to reopen communications and find mutually enjoyable activities.

◆ Alice recognized the need to spend more time with her children. With household help and some adjustments in Tim's work schedule, for awhile she was able to do this. But, as her disease worsened, this became more and more difficult. Activities like brushing her hair might take as long as half an hour. Taking a shower took the better part of two hours, and she had to sit down to do it as well as rest twice during the shower. Each of the basic routines that everyone does on a daily basis without even thinking about them, had become a monumental task. Life itself was becoming a chore.

There is no doubt that when one is suffering with illnesses that are physically exhausting or disabling, or with disabilities due to injury, it takes longer to get things done and to get going in the morning. There are many obstacles throughout the day. When persons with disabilities work, they have to get up sometimes two hours earlier to be at work on time. Sometimes the effort seems too much. Persons who have lost the use of their hands have difficulty eating, and turning pages. Many disabilities make going to the bathroom a difficult and time-consuming problem! The effort that has to go into doing these basic activities of daily living may seem overwhelming. It can be so discouraging!

Although the spontaneity in doing these tasks that normal people enjoy may be over, careful planning can allow persons with significant disability to do these chores well. In addition, many techniques and aids to speed things up and make them easier now exist.

A first step is locating and enlisting the help of public-health agencies that can send a registered nurse to the home who will evaluate needs and make recommendations. The visiting nurse can make recommendations for home health attendants to help with bathing, dressing, and cooking, can recommend equipment and ways of doing things to conserve energy, can suggest appropriate furniture rearrangements or even more appropriate uses of different rooms in the house. The nurse can also be instrumental in speeding up the processes involved in getting help or can teach how to change a dressing, or how to complete a necessary daily task of self-care (See Chapter 5: Finding and Using Community Resources.)

These situations illustrate that illness can alter relationships at any stage of life between marriage partners, parents and children, and grandparents and grandchildren, or really, between any family members. The specific illnesses cited may not apply to you, but likely, you and your family will have faced concerns similar to some of those described. Remember that regardless of the specific physical or mental illness, or the type of physical or mental limitation, the same approach can be used to deal with and cope with the emotional issues that arise.

♦ Keep communication open. Listen to each other without responding or trying to make each other feel better. *No blaming.* When talking to a family member about your feelings or thoughts, always begin with "I think" or "I feel."

♦ Recognize that former roles, such as decision-maker or breadwinner in the family, may be changed when those roles do not have to change. Make sure to discuss all necessary changes so that the ill or disabled person's role in the family is not undermined accidentally.

♦ Feelings of anger, disappointment, and fear are appropriate. Don't discount your feelings as silly or bad.

♦ Talking about the illness or disability will not upset the sick or disabled person and worsen his/her condition.

♦ Spouses must plan to do things together that they have always enjoyed doing. Sit down together and plan activities, and exactly when you are going to do them.

♦ Each family member, including the ill or disabled person, must keep involved in family decisions, work, problem solving, and activities. Sit down and explicitly assign tasks.

♦ Flag behaviors that suggest that either the ill person or family members are not actively participating in the family, and might be withdrawing.

♦ Find new roles to replace old roles.

♦ Try not to expect children to parent. Adolescent children should be allowed to develop in as normal a way as possible. They can be expected to help out but should not be expected to give up their social lives entirely.

♦ Family meetings to assign jobs, involve the ill or disabled person and children, keep communication open, and watch for changes can be very helpful. Plan these meetings each week.

CHAPTER 9

Managing Personality Changes

The physical changes and limitations imposed by illness or injury are painful for the whole family. Yet the illness may extend beyond the person's body and affect his mind as well, or in the case of Alzheimer's Disease and many other mental illnesses, the disease may primarily affect the mind. The personality and mood changes that accompany many diseases may come about for a variety of reasons that will be covered in this chapter. While such changes may not be amenable to any specific therapy, it is often easier to live with them, and it may be helpful in minimizing them, once we understand why they have come about. The vignettes in this chapter include Len and Megan, a young couple in which the man has had a stroke, and an alteration of his personality because of it; Glenn and Ann, which illustrates an example of medication causing personality change; and Bonita, in which early problems of Alzheimer's Disease are discussed.

Len and Megan

◆ Len had a stroke at age thirty-three. While shaving one morning, he suddenly lost his speech and became weak on the right side. Since he was a young child, Len had known he had a hole in his heart, but he had lived a totally normal life and rarely thought about his heart. The doctors determined that the stroke was caused by a small clot that went from the heart and plugged a small artery in Len's brain, but within a few hours he seemed to be completely back to normal again; except for the need to take a medication to keep his blood from clotting, he resumed his previous life-style.

Len's wife, Megan, however, noticed soon after the stroke that Len was a different person. At first she could not quite figure out the difference, but then she realized that problem-solving tasks he had done easily before the stroke now took him much longer; where he used to spend hours repairing appliances and machines about the house, he now became quickly frustrated and gave up. He was not as much fun as he used to be either! He had always had a temper but rarely showed it, and never flew into a rage in public. Since the stroke, she found him yelling at other drivers on the road; he once insulted a waiter, and they were asked to leave a restaurant; and he yelled at the kids so often that they were avoiding him altogether. Worst of all, he had been told by his boss that he would have to control his temper better, or he would be fired. Megan felt almost as if she were living with a stranger.

In many ways Len is a stranger, not only to Megan, but also to himself. These subtle changes, which may be a result of the stroke, certainly startle and concern him as much as they do the people around him. Frequently the stroke victim has lost control over the outbursts which cause him embarrassment and guilt. When dexterity tasks, which were easy to perform before the stroke, become hard or impossible to do, this causes fear as well as frustration. Embarrassment about losses, and fear about loss of control and the inability to manage, can frequently result in the stroke victim trying to hide or deny these changes. Further, anger and resentment over the alienation of friends and family make things even worse. Len and his family may well start to feel vulnerable and frightened. Because of the social problems this is causing, they will also soon become isolated.

It is important to try to determine whether the changes in behavior are related to the stroke, related to medication, or related to emotional reactions to the illness. Sometimes feelings of depression and anxiety can explain the behavior. It is not uncommon to feel fear and anxiety after suffering a life-threatening illness. Anticipating negative changes in life-style as well as new feelings of vulnerability, can result in depression and anxiety about the future. Anger can then result and lead to outbursts. However, a stroke can also leave a person with permanent losses that result in losses of dexterity as well as exaggerations of previous personality traits. As in Len's case, previous loss of temper can be exaggerated after a stroke and cause embarrassment, not only to the family but also to Len. Frequently, men in Len's position feel very guilty about this explosiveness. In either case, consultation with a professional who is familiar with behavioral problems associated with strokes, is recommended (see Chapter 5: Finding and Using Community Resources). When loss of control is a factor as in Len's case, there are behavioral techniques which might help him reestablish a sense of control. For example, Len is easily angered. Teaching him relaxation training techniques, and when to use them through behavioral or biofeedback treatment, can help him to gain control over his anger prior to the explosiveness. Reducing the anger eliminates the explosiveness and restores a sense of control to Len. Relaxation training has also been very helpful in reducing hypertension. This technique reduces arousal levels and helps reduce stress and anxiety.

There are several types of relaxation training. In some cases, such as with cancer patients after they have begun chemotherapy, imagery techniques are used to reduce anxiety and help with feelings of nausea, which sometimes precede chemotherapy treatment after it has begun. The scenes used in the guided imagery are usually of places that are fondly thought of as relaxing to the person, or known to have a calming effect. The second method used in relaxation training is the progressive tensing and relaxing of each muscle from all the muscle groups in the body. The contrast between experiencing the tension sensations, and then letting go and experiencing the relaxation sensations, teaches the person the difference between tensed and relaxed muscles. A person cannot be both tensed and relaxed at the same time. As the person learns how to notice which muscles are tensed, he or she can think about loosening that muscle and be able to do so. Then he or she can scan him/herself during the day and relax tensed muscles. In the process of concentrating on these muscles and in relaxing them,

BUILDING A NEW DREAM

tension, anger, and anxiety are reduced. The progressive relaxation of each muscle group brings a calming effect.

First, the therapist asks the client to sit in a chair as comfortably as possible. The person closes his/her eyes and tries to get comfortable. Then the therapist directs the client to ". . . concentrate on your breathing. Breathe in and out and just concentrate on your breathing. Let all other thoughts leave your mind for a while and only concentrate on your breathing. Now I want you to clench your right fist. Clench it and notice the tension. Study the tension and now relax your fist, let the muscles in your right hand get loose, and notice the difference between the tension and relaxation. . . ." The therapist continues using all the various muscle groups throughout the body. There are also a number of audiotapes utilizing relaxation training techniques available in some of the larger bookstores, which can guide a person through the maneuvers of progressive muscle relaxation. Some tapes use imagery to teach deep relaxation.

Relaxation techniques have also been used in pain management. Chronic pain, which results from illnesses such as arthritis or disability, is a constant factor for the ill or disabled. Constant pain interferes with relationships, and alters the personality of the ill or disabled person. Experiencing pain all the time can result in social isolation and in loss of time at work. Relaxation techniques can help to reduce the experience of pain by reducing the anxiety and tension that frequently accompany attacks of pain, and because of the deep concentration and calming effects. The danger of addiction and negative side effects make the constant use of medication to control pain problematic. Therefore, relaxation skills, meditation, and self-hypnosis are often good tools to use to help manage pain. Professionals trained in these behavior therapy techniques can be consulted for training in any of these modalities. There are also pain clinics that use these techniques and biofeedback to help people manage pain.

Discussions with a professional about ways that Megan can work with Len during these times foster cooperative problem solving. For example, Megan can remind Len to begin the relaxation techniques when she sees him working himself up, and when they are in situations that she knows excite him.

Permanent changes in Len's personality do place a big stress on the relationship. Often one hears family members say that the ill person is not trying, because if they really wanted to they would be different. This frequently is the family members' way of trying to cope with the permanency of the changes and the sense that nothing can be done. A personality problem is often more difficult for the family and the ill person to cope with also, because the defect is not physically visible. This, along with the fact that emotional illness is even less acceptable in our society than physical illness, greatly confounds their ability to grapple with the problem.

Associations of persons with the same illness are a good source of support. The American Heart Association sponsors heart clubs, held at hospitals, which offer monthly meeetings to help families handle the impact of strokes on the individual and the family. Sharing concerns with others can lead to learning how to handle some of the similar problems that each family experiences.

Glenn and Ann

◆ Glenn had worked for General Motors for forty years when he retired at age sixty-five. He was very proud of his long career there and liked going to work every day. He and his wife Ann had looked forward to his retirement, but Glenn soon found himself lost without his work and the camaraderie of the other workers. It was not long before the symptoms of peptic ulcer disease that he had had as a young man started to bother him again. His doctor put him on some tablets which seemed to help a lot.

Ann had been distressed at Glenn's poor adaptation to retirement, but she became really frightened soon after he started on the treatment for his ulcer. He became listless and lethargic. He seemed just to watch TV all day, and she often found him asleep in front of the set; in conversations they had, he was forgetful and could not seem to concentrate on anything. She was afraid the idleness of his retirement was causing him to lose his mind, and she felt helpless.

Frequently, side effects of medication can cause symptoms that resemble depression—listlessness, forgetfulness, and sleepiness. Whenever medication is being taken, it is very important to check with the physician about possible side effects. Even if retirement is difficult for Glenn, and he is having some emotional reaction about reaching this stage in his life, he could also be reacting to medication side effects. These things can coexist. The reactions to the medication, however, can make the apparent reactions to the life changes seem as if they were much worse than they might actually be. It is very important to check this out. No matter what else seems to be going on, it is important to determine if the medication is causing side effects. If it is, there are often alternative medications which can be prescribed. When there is an acute medical problem or in cases when there are many medications being taken at the same time, as with many elderly patients, certain medications could be stopped, since they may not be needed. This can prevent problems with interactive effects between medications. Today it is often not necessary to depend on only one medication, and medication changes are easily made in consultation with your physician.

◆ With great relief, Ann watched Glenn's mind clear considerably after his medication was changed. And, thankfully, the other medication seemed to be taking care of his ulcer as well as the original one! However, after several weeks, Ann still felt Glenn was not back to normal. He still spent much more time watching TV than he had done before, and she sometimes found him asleep in the middle of the afternoon, which was very unlike him.

After the medication side effects are checked, the negative effects of the medication should be able to be reduced or eliminated by changing the dosage, or changing to another medication. Personality changes that remain probably relate to the underlying depression arising from Glenn's difficulties in adjusting to his retirement. Mood changes are one of many personality changes that signal depression.

Retirement may mean more time for travel and leisure-time

activities, but it also means a drastic change in the way time is spent. Work satisfies many human needs, such as the need for productivity, achievement, power, influence, and usefulness. Loss of job-related status and income can bring on additional stress and make it harder to adjust to being home. Work provides a structure to one's day and a social setting. How much the amount of structure and need for a social network with others will affect the reaction to retirement, depends on people's personalities. Whether retirement was planned for and anticipated, or forced, also affects adjustment. If a person is used to finding little chores and projects to do at home, retirement can be seen as a time to finish the hundreds of projects one starts and doesn't complete, or can't even start for lack of time. On the other hand, a person who lived for his work, had few hobbies, and is not handy about the house may find himself anxious and dissatisfied. Dissatisfaction with unstructured time may only become a problem after retirement when one finds oneself with a lot of unstructured time to fill. Further, retirement frequently leaves many folks feeling that time has really moved on, and that there is not much time left. It is important to know that feelings about time passing are normal and usual. Feeling influential and needed are also important feelings to regain, and new activities need to replace old ones so that these feelings can be rekindled. Anger is not an unusual result of feeling a loss of role, and loss of a social network. Glenn, without direction or structure and the usual tasks of his work day, may be feeling aimless and disgruntled. Ann may be having her own difficulties getting used to her schedule now that Glenn is home. Many couples make the role changes that retirement brings; however, in some cases, there is a need to acknowledge the feelings of loss, and work at planning specific activities and reformulating goals. If the conflicts become prolonged or depressed symptoms worsen, couples' counseling could help resolve these conflicts, and help couples find new interests and activities to do together.

Bonita

◆ Bonita's husband died of a heart attack when they were both fifty-five. It had never been a very satisfying marriage, and after the death, Bonita seemed to blossom. She began to take some classes at the local college, developed a whole new set of friends, and joined a tennis club. Then when Bonita was age sixty-two, her daughter Elaine began to notice some disturbing changes in her mother. She was beginning to lose her energy and feistiness. Her friends were complaining that she was not showing up for tennis dates, and when she did, could not seem to concentrate on the games. She seemed unable to keep her mind on one thing, and was not much fun to be around anymore. Yet Elaine knew of nothing that had happened to her mother, or any reason why she should be unhappy or depressed. Life had been the best it had ever been for Bonita!

Personality changes as a result of small strokes in the brain unnoticed or undiagnosed, or because of Alzheimer's Disease, or other neurologic problems, are extremely devastating to both the person and family members.

Fears about losses of memory and what that may mean, often result in family members constantly correcting the affected family member. Family members begin to get irritated over the repetition and forgetfulness. Their irritation is usually related to the difficulty they are having coping with these personality changes in someone they love. There is a real need and a desire to believe that the person they love can be themselves again, if they would just concentrate or try. Of course, that is not going to happen, and the sooner the family members realize this, the less frustration and alienation there will be.

◆ Bonita and Elaine had really come to enjoy each other's company in the last few years. They frequently ate out together, or Bonita invited Elaine over for home-cooked meals that would often be followed by a lively discussion about politics, or some other timely subject. Elaine came to know and appreciate many things about her mother that she had been totally oblivious to when she was growing up. Bonita had always been a meticulous housekeeper, and gourmet cooking had been her hobby. Recently, however, whenever Elaine visited, she noticed that the dusting was not done, and sometimes things were lying around, and the dishes from the day before were not washed. A few times lately, Bonita had invited Elaine for dinner and then completely forgotten about it. She even forgot what she had ordered when they went out to a restaurant! The lively discussions were now a thing of the past. Elaine had tried initiating some, but in the past few weeks she found Bonita repeating the same sentence several times, and then completely losing her train of thought. It was painful for both to hear. Something terrible was happening to Bonita!

Frequently for people like Bonita, the realization that they are forgetting things, and that it is getting worse, is very frightening. The fear and sense of helplessness often result in apathy and withdrawal. These changes add to the fear and sadness of the family. The fight seems gone, and often the apathy leads to neglect of family responsibilities that always were so important to the person. For example, Bonita is no longer as concerned about cleaning the house. Dinners that used to be waiting for her daughter whenever she came to visit, are not cooked. Many of these changes reflect Bonita's increasing loss of short-term memory, a hallmark of Alzheimer's Disease. What seems so frightening is that the person whom everyone was used to and loved, seems to be gone, though her physical body is not and serves as a constant reminder of the loss. It is not fun to be with her anymore. Elaine can feel very guilty about not enjoying her mother as well as very sad. Not only does she have to begin the mourning process, but she also has to watch her mother get progressively worse. Her mother may get so debilitated that Elaine will also have to face questions about home care or nursing homes. In the meantime, If Elaine and her mother can openly communicate their concerns, and talk together about what would be helpful, this could reduce a lot of the fears for them both. This does not necessarily make the stricken person feel worse, or result in embarrassing or saddening them, which is frequently the concern. It does allow planning for the future. If nothing is said, then they are all alone with the realization that some awful changes are happening. When there is open communication and sharing of feelings, there can also be planning, and then the feelings of being all alone are lessened; they can also share their grief. In addition, before it is impossible, discussions can be held about the future and what Bonita would like her future to be. Sometimes people want to write a living will, or plan for burial sites or nursing homes. There can be added peace and relief if these conversations are held, even though they are sad and difficult.

Alzheimer's Disease and other problems that result in memory losses and personality changes, leave everyone feeling so helpless. Open communication among family members, memory techniques, and planning can take some of that feeling of helplessness away. However, there are some practical aids that can be used to allow an afflicted person to function independently as long as possible, and help the caretaker. For example:

◆ Make labels for drawers stating what is in each drawer so that the person can easily find clothes in the bedroom or utensils in the kitchen.

◆ Make signs, e.g., "Take Shower" or "Turn Off Water," to remind the person to do things and post them in unavoidable places.

◆ Keep a large calendar handy on which the activities of the day can be written. Remembering what day it is may be difficult, but this kind of information is always available from listening to the radio in the morning.

◆ Hire household help as the ill person worsens to prolong the period of independence and the eventual caretaker's independence.

A good guide for persons and families coping with Alzheimer's Disease is *The 36-Hour Day,* by Nancy L. Mace and Peter V. Rabins, M.D. This book offers many suggestions for managing behavioral changes in persons with Alzheimer's Disease and related diseases.

There are also Alzheimer's Disease support groups for families and friends, run by self-help organizations and hospitals. As with other illnesses or disabilities, there is a national organization, the Alzheimer's Disease and Related Disorders Association, which through local groups in some communities provides education and family support. In Canada, the local chapters of the Alzheimer Association or the Alzheimer Society, should be contacted. It is very helpful to contact these groups and meet with other family members with whom you can talk. Learning about ways to cope with Alzheimer's Disease, as well as learning about such matters as research findings, home health aides, legislation, and insurance coverage, etc., can provide the social support that can lessen the trauma of Alzheimer's Disease on the family.

◆ Some illnesses can cause personality changes. These changes may be embarrassing to the whole family. Professional consultation for relaxation, and behavioral feedback techniques may help the person to control socially unacceptable behaviors.

◆ Medications can cause sleepiness and other mood swings. When these occur, all medications the person takes should be reviewed by his physician. Any that might cause these changes should be discontinued if possible.

◆ Reactions to illness, like depression, can also cause personality changes. When this degree of depression exists, professional counseling is often necessary.

◆ In dementing diseases like Alzheimer's Disease, family members can talk about the problems and plan for the future. They should try to maintain the person's independence as long as possible.

◆ Helping keep the ill person as independent as possible, participating in disease-related organizations, and meeting other people who are experiencing similar problems can be very helpful in lessening the trauma of the disease on the family.

CHAPTER 10

Preventing Emotional Exhaustion

Inevitably, the entire attention of a family becomes directed at the ill person when disease or disability strikes. How central a role that disease will play in the ongoing life of that family, depends on how the family collectively and individually learns to manage the demands and uncertainties of the illness. Learning to recognize and cope with some predictable situations will greatly facilitate and speed up the family's ability to successfully coexist with the unwelcome new illness.

One of the situations that can be a part of almost any ongoing illness is emotional exhaustion. Of course, the ill person can experience this through the ravages of the disability or disease itself, or through frustration at not being the same person he was before. However, it is as likely that other family members will become burnt-out by the illness, even to the extent that it destroys their lives and disrupts their family.

Emotional exhaustion can come from a well partner taking on the entire burden of an illness after a spouse's heart attack, as in the Mel and Margot vignette; or it can come from bending to unreasonable demands of the ill person, especially an ill child, as in the case of Alexandra, who has asthma. Sometimes taking on the personal care of the affected person can be overwhelming and disrupt multiple family members, as in the vignette of the middle-aged couple, Karl and Nancy, who struggle with the effects of Parkinson's Disease. And, finally, exhaustion can come from well-intentioned but misdirected intervention by relatives or others outside the immediate family, which is discussed in the vignette of Hugo and Rachel, a couple coping with MS. These vignettes demonstrate how the problems can occur and be manifested in a variety of ways, how they can be recognized by those affected, and how they might be handled.

Mel and Margot

◆ Mel and Margot had been married for ten years and had one child, Michael, age six. Mel had a "type A" personality and, as is typical of such people, rose through the ranks in a local ceramic tile manufacturing firm to become the operations manager. At age forty-three he was in charge of the general operations of the firm and directly responsible for 123 people. His perfectionistic personality led him to work fourteen-hour days. Margot had gotten used to this and adapted to his devotion to his job and the little time spent with the family. One morning, he awakened feeling as if he had the flu but Mel, being who he was, went to work anyway. At ten o'clock, Margot received a call from the local hospital that her husband had been brought in with a massive heart attack. On arrival at the hospital, she learned that his heart had stopped twice and his chance of survival was less than fifty percent.

Mel survived, but the damage to his heart was severe, and he developed an enlarged heart and chronic heart failure. Over the next few months, it became clear he would not be able to return to his job as he became quickly fatigued, retained water easily, and occasionally had chest pains even with medication.

Margot had had a very productive and satisfying career of her own as a special education teacher. Now her role as the sole breadwinner enhanced the importance of her work. Yet Margot was becoming very frustrated. Her field was one of constant change and to keep up with recent advances, she had to read journals and participate in workshops. It was becoming very difficult for her to do this. When she came home at night, the housekeeper who cared for Michael went home, and Margot was expected to start all over again. She had to make dinner, play with Michael, take care of any needs her husband had, and get everything ready for the next day. To make matters worse, it seemed that anything she did was not quite good enough for Mel. He did not like the food, her hair wasn't styled properly, she did not give the housekeeper adequate instructions . . . Margot began to hate coming home at night. She was really working an eighteen-hour day and was constantly tired. She had no time for herself or to keep current in her career. She began to resent her husband, possibly even hate him; at the least she knew he could be doing more than lying on the couch all day, feeling sorry for himself.

This problem actually began when Margot agreed to do all that she is doing. Although her husband's schedule must be decidedly different than prior to his heart attack, he can participate more than it seems they have expected of him. Margot's expectations for herself, as well as for her husband, need to be realistic. It is not realistic to expect yourself to work full time, take care of your young child, cook, and care for your ill husband. Trying to do all these things can lead to emotional exhaustion. A common consequence of a serious illness is that expectations for contribution by the ill person to the various needs of the family is subconsciously lowered by both persons. Mel can cook and, most likely, do other family chores around the house. When Margot gets home, she needs some quiet time for herself, even if it is just half an hour to shower, or sit down by herself.

Margot has to be careful that guilt and other feelings about her freedom, about separation from her child, and guilt about her good health, does not cause her to take on additional and unnecessary work which results in feelings of anger and resentment. Mel's unhappiness is also being expressed through his complaints and dissatisfaction. Margot is not in a position to sympathize. Lowered expectations for him and poor planning for extra help contribute to both their feelings of unhappiness. In this case, it would be a great help to have the housekeeper live in or stay through dinner. Though the circumstances in each family are somewhat different, it is often possible to reduce the burden on the well person considerably by making relatively minor adjustments in the existing structure.

Mel's unhappiness may be reflecting his own sense that he is a burden. He needs opportunities to share in their life and participate in the activities around him. Rather than criticizing Margot for giving instructions to the housekeeper, he might give them himself. This will help both Margot and Mel to reestablish a sense of independence. They both had careers that they had been free to pursue and enjoy. It is just as important for the well spouse to be able to return to those activities that gave him/her a sense of personal self-worth and accomplishment, as it is for the physically ill person to maintain some control and the sense that he is still needed in the family. Mel was a very career-oriented man, and the loss must be very difficult for him. As with many men or women who are in a position of considerable responsibility and then fall ill, Mel may have a need to regain some independence. Under the present circumstances, neither of them can respond to this. Mel is underfunctioning, and as long as Margot overfunctions for him, he will continue to lie on the couch all day. It is possible also that Mel is experiencing anger and other feelings about his lost career. Mel's apathy and his demands on his wife suggest something unspoken is going on in his mind.

Two things would be helpful. Margot and her husband have to find some time to sit down together and talk about their current situation. Margot may have kept silent in the past when she was unhappy with her husband's behavior, but now she can no longer be silent as she is in danger of becoming emotionally exhausted. Mel and Margot need to talk about the work that Mel can now do either at home or in the community to feel productive. Margot can open up the subject by telling her husband that she is exhausted. Then she can suggest that they find out exactly what the limitations on Mel's activities really have to be. The first step here might have to be a trip to his physician to find out just exactly what level of activity he can tolerate. It may be that both Mel and Margot are operating on the erroneous assumption that Mel's activity needs to be severely limited, or alternatively maybe it does. Even in this circumstance, there are usually many sedentary jobs that could tap his interest and former intrinsic enjoyment of work. Secondly, to take the domestic load off of Margot—which is essentially a second full-time job at present—as suggested in the paragraph above, Mel and Margot need to rearrange their home-care with the housekeeper or make other home-care decisions. The arrangement in which the housekeeper stays through dinner, for example, allows Margot the time she needs to herself when she gets home. She can shower, read the newspaper, put her child to bed, or whatever she wishes, and then she and Mel can sit and spend some time together.

If Mel can share some of the family duties and Margot can feel that life is not so much harder now that she has to give up all her activities, each person can feel that they can function, despite the impact of the illness. This then allows them to begin to cope with the changes in their lives and feel hopeful about the future.

Even in families where the burden of the illness is not as oppressive as in this vignette, emotional exhaustion often occurs. It can creep up insidiously as increasing irritation by one or both partners, growing resentment of the sick role of the ill person, and a suspicion on the part of the over-burdened well person that the ill person is not really as disabled as he/she makes out to be. Be on the lookout for these danger signs! If they occur, sit down, and think about and talk about ways in which some of the burden can be shifted off of the well person(s) who are shouldering it.

◆ Mel and Margot hired a housekeeper. With her help and Mel's taking on of some household tasks, the family was able to manage better, though Margot still had to make an effort to allow enough time for herself and time to spend with Michael. Then, just when things seemed to have settled down, Mel developed pneumonia. This stress, on top of his already damaged heart, caused heart failure and Mel had to be hospitalized. Now Margot had to stop at the hospital every evening after work, as well as take on the jobs Mel was doing and find time for Michael. Furthermore, the doctors had told them that Mel might never fully recover and would be more limited than before. After four days of this, Margot was ready to scream. She found herself at one moment thinking it might be better if he were to die, and at the next moment unable to believe that she could have such thoughts. How could she survive?

It is hard to believe that anything else could happen to make the job of caring for a person with a chronic illness or disability harder. When there is a medical emergency, however, that is precisely what happens. It is like *déjà vu* to the time the illness first appeared. The same soul-searching to understand why this is happening, and the feelings of grief and unfairness all reappear. Margot needs support. It is not possible to handle all of this alone; no one need be that brave or courageous. Margot's thoughts that it would be better if Mel died, are natural at a time when she feels like she does not know how she is going to survive. It is a frightening time, and she will feel scared and alone. It feels to her as if she simply cannot handle anything more; she is exhausted.

Margot needs to ask for specific help. She needs to call friends, if friends do not offer their help. Friends or family members can visit Mel in the hospital to relieve Margot several nights a week. Friends can take Michael for the weekend, or even for a week so that Margot can attend to the insurance, hospital, and medical needs of Mel. (See Chapter 4: Anticipating Medical Crises.) Friends or family members can stay with her so that cooking needs and Michael's needs can be met while she has to be at the hospital.

Family and friends need to let Margot ventilate and talk about her feelings. This is a very sad time, and it feels like the same tragedy all over again. This is not a time to ask her to be strong and not be emotional.

This new crisis may bring added financial burdens on the family and may leave Mel more disabled than before. To get through this new problem, planning is essential. Margot needs to meet with Mel's doctor as soon as possible to get a feeling of what Mel's status is likely to be after he recovers from this illness, and whether he will need more assistance and support than before. She needs to plan how she will manage when he comes home, if his needs are different from before. It may be necessary to call community agencies for advice and recommendations, and to reserve additional help if this looks likely. If financial burdens will result from this, she should contact social workers who will help her get in touch with the proper resources. If she waits until Mel is discharged to do this, his early days at home may be very difficult, and she may become even more exhausted.

Margot may need to speak to friends or family about help with new financial problems that the hospitalization or Mel's immobilization have brought about and help in filling out insurance papers, etc. Again, this is the time for Margot to ask for what she needs and not to feel that she has to bear it all herself. Her needs are valid, and getting them met is essential to the entire family's well being.

The destabilizing effect of this emergency throws the whole family back into crisis. Afterwards there is a new level of fear, sadness, and disillusionment—instead of getting better, things are getting worse; these feelings are natural and are often unavoidable. If the family does not eventually stabilize emotionally again, it may be helpful to seek counseling.

Alexandra

◆ Alexandra was the second of two daughters in the Praxton family. Unlike her robust sister, she had always been small and thin and had some eczema, but was otherwise well until she developed asthma at age six. Alexandra's asthma was quite mild in the beginning, and while it was frightening to have difficulty breathing, she responded well to medication. Her disease worsened over the next few years, and she required several hospitalizations; several times her mother was afraid she might stop breathing. Alexandra's family was terrified of this possibility and, after the first such episode, remodeled their lives to accommodate the illness. Mrs. Praxton quit her job to be home with Alexandra; the family moved to a drier climate. Alexandra's asthma attacks had a strong emotional component, and she often got her way to prevent her from having a severe asthma attack. Because of Alexandra's illness, her sister Mina was expected to take care of Alexandra. If Alexandra aggravated Mina and a fight ensued, Alexandra would often develop an asthma attack, and Mina would be severely punished. In fact, Mina felt that most of the time her parents spent with her was criticizing or punishing her; she had given up her friends when they moved; she had given up her pet cat because Alex was allergic to it; she had even given up her room for her sister, whom she considered a brat.

Nothing will exhaust a family more than the guilt and responsibility that a child's illness can place on them. The danger is that the family will make all their individual and family decisions, based only on what is best for the ill child. The family members can become enveloped in the myth that if any member pursues his own needs or interests, he will be responsible for endangering the ill sibling's well being. This myth becomes so terrorizing that siblings of the ill child may not be able to lead normal lives as separate, healthy children, but rather can be tied to satisfying the demands of the ill child. Often mothers and fathers believe that being good parents means ensuring that everyone must sacrifice and dote on the ill child. They think it is their responsibility to their ill child. This leads to overprotectiveness and deprives these children of the security of an environment in which they are treated normally, and in which they can feel they are controlled and safe.

Rather than being beneficial to the ill child, special treatment of the type Alexandra has had can be very detrimental to her ultimate emotional health. She, unfortunately, has been treated as so helpless and as such an invalid that she must see herself as dependent and incapable of living her own life.

Mina cannot help but resent her sister. In the long run, she may feel that she also had a disabling illness, because so many decisions in her life and her relationships were determined by her sister's needs. Mina's own separate needs have been sacrificed for her sister's. The result is that she becomes, along with the rest of the family, emotionally exhausted trying to meet her sister's needs and demands. One of the most unfortunate of all of the long-term effects of this type of treatment of an ill child, is that the well siblings may grow up with severe emotional handicaps, and may have difficulty in their relationships.

Sometimes families get caught up in a cycle of guilt and manipulation. In this situation, one or more family members, often the mother or a sibling, will feel responsible for the child's illness, and the guilt associated with this will feed into the child's unwarranted power in the family and allow his manipulation. This sort of guilt is often seen in hereditary illnesses, like cystic fibrosis or in accidents resulting in long-term disability. It is possible in the case of injury that someone in the family was partially responsible for the injury, and this makes the situation even more difficult. Nevertheless, much more harm than good and much more emotional turmoil will result from allowing the child to be the center of all family decisions. While having a child with special needs will always have an impact on family plans, the lives and autonomy of the other family members must never be sacrificed.

One of the major mistakes that has been made in Alexandra's family and that is often made in families where guilt is a factor, is that she has been given far too much power in the family. In this example, she has been reinforced and as a result helped to learn how to manipulate the family. This detrimental use of power has to make her feel very frightened, and in turn, insecure and guilty herself. Her feelings are never expressed verbally. Any affection and attention that she gets is always centered around her attacks, thereby reinforcing her illness and giving her secondary gains because of her symptoms. This encourages her to maintain the symptoms.

Asthma, like a number of common chronic childhood diseases, is manageable and frequently is outgrown. However, Alexandra has little reason to improve. Normal expectations for her and limit setting are essential if she and her family are to lead a normal life. Families who get caught in this eventually stop living their individual lives. They become frozen in time. Time has stood still since the child's illness became a threatening part of their lives. In twenty years, when the child is grown and essentially well, the emotional impact and crippling that results from allowing this sort of behavior is likely to have left an indelible mark on family members. The disease will still be very real, and an enduring facet of their lives, even though the child might not have suffered from asthma in ten years. In these families, it is not unusual to see members still cry whenever they talk about the illness, although the child is now an adult.

Such sacrifices on the part of the child by the family are almost never warranted, and almost always result in dysfunctional coping and adaptation to the illness or injury. Harm is done to everyone. The ill child never learns to make a life for himself/herself that includes family, children, and work. The rest of the family give up their lives and forfeit their autonomy. Everyone pours all their emotional strength into the ramifications of the illness, and there is nothing left over for anything else.

To prevent this from happening, the family has to do two things. First, teach the child and appropriate caretakers how to manage the illness calmly and responsibly. Asthma and most other illnesses are controllable most of the time. Children can learn how to treat themselves when they begin to feel an attack coming on. The degree of panic they experience usually reflects the degree of panic in the household. Parents need to be calm and work with the child to manage each episode.

Also parents, the child, and appropriate siblings should talk together with the child's physician to learn about all current medications and the correct way to use them. In asthma, for example, learning how to comply and not overuse inhalers, is important in correct management. They can learn from the physician what the child has to avoid in the home and in community environments (religious, school, parks, friends' homes), to protect him/herself from precipitating substances. There is no need for this illness to get out of control. Inevitably, children need to talk about their thoughts and feelings. It is not uncommon for children with asthma to feel depressed and anxious over their illness. Not being able to breathe is terrifying and arouses fears about dying. Many children with asthma and other chronic illnesses fear they will die. It is reasonable to reassure children that they can manage this illness and won't die. As they learn how to manage acute episodes, they will gain confidence. Beginning at an age when they can first follow directions, they should be given increasing responsibility for managing medications and other aspects of the illness. This gives them a sense of control over the illness and confidence. And confidence about this is the first step to gaining mastery over the disease and allowing them to live as normal a life as possible. This is true for many illnesses like diabetes that requires insulin injections and cystic fibrosis, which requires regular medication and often chest physiotherapy. Children can also learn to manage many of these interventions for themselves.

Second, after the child has learned as best he can how to manage the illness, the most important thing to do is to treat the child like a normal child, and in the same manner as all other children are treated in the family. Siblings need to know about the illness also and how to help their brother or sister if an attack occurs, but they should not be asked to take care of their brother or sister in any unusual way. Siblings need opportunities to talk also. They often feel fearful that their brother or sister might die, and they may feel guilty that they are not the sick one. Siblings also have to know that while some precautions might have to be taken in the home, for the most part, they can lead their lives normally. For example, in this vignette, Mina could have been told that although she could not have the cat anymore, she could have something else. Her parents could let her pick out an appropriate pet and go with her to buy it. She might not be able to have a pet cat, but she could have some tropical fish.

Siblings fight, and they also help each other out. If one child is always blamed in a fight, the other one knows immediately that that will happen and uses it. This just instills hatred between siblings. If a fight ensues and an asthmatic attack follows, treat the attack as separate from the fight, and manage it as it has always been managed no matter what the cause. Often, specific causes for the asthmatic attacks are not known. Do not blame the fight or other children for the attack. Let siblings live their lives and pay attention to them. Go to their school and after-school events. Take interest in their development also.

It is easy to become preoccupied with the sick child. Parents might find it helpful to monitor themselves to make sure that they are not doing that. You might work out a system where each parent checks the other weekly to make sure they are spending time with each child and not neglecting, overusing, or taking the well child for granted.

Parents should not give up things in their lives either, for illness in a child, unless it is truly medically necessary. It is not necessary, for example, for a parent to quit a job, if they were not planning to anyway and there is no medical indication from their physician that they need to be home. Staying home with an asthmatic child because he/she has asthma and not because it is medically indicated, may be sending messages to the child that there is reason to be afraid, because the parent is afraid and that they need special attention. If a child is going to be left with a relative, housekeeper, or baby-sitter after school hours and before a parent gets home, then that caretaker should be one who can learn how to handle the illness, and he/she can be taught how to handle medication, or any other situation that might arise. The main thing is to make sure he/she is comfortable with the illness and knows what to do in an acute or emergency situation. If caretakers are having a difficult time—parents, grandparents, and other family members, who justifiably have many questions and concerns when a child has a chronic illness—then they need to talk with friends, family, or professionals, to help them overcome their fears and guilt, and get parenting advice.

Parents who are having difficulty knowing how to respond to their ill child and to other siblings in the family, might find it helpful to read books or literature on the subject, or join support groups run through the American Lung Association and by self-help or-ganizations in the community. Call the local chapter of American Lung Association in your community if your child has asthma, for example, and ask for literature and the names of clubs, support groups, or other parents so you can ask questions, find out how other parents manage with their asthmatic children, and share experiences and information. In some communities, the American Lung Association offers a Family Asthma Program designed for asthmatic children and their families. Be sure to see if a Family Asthma Program exists in your community, and go to at least one meeting. You don't have to commit yourself to long-term atten-dance, but give yourself a chance to check things out and ask questions. The American Diabetes Association also has support groups for parents, children, and young adults. Cystic Fibrosis Associations exist in nearly all communities. These associations can be extremely helpful. Go to the library, or look in the phone book to locate the associations in your community. (See Appendix 1.)

Karl and Nancy

◆ Parkinson's Disease was not unfamiliar to Karl, as his uncle had had it for many years before his death. In fact, he suspected that Nancy might have it even before the diagnosis was made on her fifty-second birthday. He had recognized her difficulty in getting up from the bed and the problem in initiating her steps, and he had noted the mild, but new, rolling tremor of her fingers as she sat watching TV. He did not, however, have any sense of how the disease would progress over the next few years. The doctors had told Karl and Nancy that it would gradually get worse, but that they would try to control the symptoms with medication. Karl and Nancy were reassured by this, but what actually happened over the next five years had all the security of walking through an enemy minefield. Nancy had many side effects from her medication, and at unpredictable times, experienced wild and bizarre movements of her arms and face. Even worse, her disease progressed more rapidly than predicted, and her ability to walk and write were impaired. At times, the doctors seemed to find just the right combination of medications, and she would be almost normal for a while; then without warning, the disease would seem to break through, and she would be worse than before.

Karl and Nancy's son, Ricky, had been in his sophomore year of college when Nancy became ill. Ricky had continued on with his studies, but had been distraught with what was happening at home. His formerly organized, competent, and confident father was at loose ends. He had aged ten years in the past two. He had been up for a major promotion in the insurance firm he worked for, but had lost it, because he did not have the energy to do the necessary paperwork. To Ricky, this disease seemed to consume his father's life as well as his mother's; his father no longer spoke of the sailboat he had planned to build when he retired. In fact, he hardly did anything but care for his wife anymore. Ricky decided he had better go home and help out before his father became ill as well. He could finish college later.

Often with diseases that follow a progressive course, families become very focused on the ill person, and controlled by the episodic nature of the illness. Because there is no stabilization, the family members feel they cannot continue with their lives. Kevin's father is a good example. Men and women in their fifties are often at the peak of their career paths. Kevin's father gave up perhaps twenty years of building toward the higher salary and responsibilities this promotion meant. But more important, he gave up his needs and the personal sense of accomplishment it would have meant.

In addition, he is giving up his interests. Sailing provided him with an opportunity to relax and renew his energy. Under the misguided impression that his wife's illness requires him to give up all his needs and autonomy, he is making sacrifices which will cause him emotional exhaustion and burn-out. The result could well be that he will grow to resent his wife and begin to treat her cruelly. This will in turn cause him great guilt and shame. Often, family members reason that when the disease gets a little worse, they will get an attendant or nurse to help with the care of the sick person; then they devote increasing amounts of their time to that care as the disease insidiously progresses. It is very critical that families not wait for the disease to progress; when spouses and children notice that they are beginning to have difficulty maintaining their usual duties at work, or when they begin to give up hobbies and satisfying leisure activities, it is time to organize help. It is vital not to become enslaved to the disease under the misguided feeling that only you can provide adequate care. Even if the sick person expects you to provide all the care, that is not reasonable or in either of your best interests. It is important to resume goals and plans that were in progress before the onset of the illness.

Ricky is about to make the same mistakes as his father. Ricky is at a point in his own personal development that requires him to gain independence from his family, and complete his education so that he can begin his own career path. Often children who return home when there is no acute or immediate crisis find it very hard to leave again, and many never marry or leave home. The family colludes in this and rather than encouraging Ricky, for example, to pursue his own life as they should, they might tacitly encourage him to stay home and help. Often well-meaning relatives or friends see this as a necessary sacrifice, and refer to the family members and siblings who have sacrificed their lives as wonderful children.

In certain circumstances, children can and need to be called on to help, but this must be done with a balance in mind. Ricky can always be called on to respond in crises or emergencies, but he is grown now and separated from home, and must pursue his own life goals. If he returns home for an indefinite period and sacrifices his schooling, he may eventually become resentful, angry, and depressed. Family members must be careful that when they are feeling needy and frightened, they do not inadvertently encourage the children to come home and stay at the expense of their own development and maturation.

It is reasonable for Ricky to help his father by aiding him in finding a way to get some help. It is important for Karl, through pursuing his own social activities, to get a respite from the emotionally draining daily demands of caring for Nancy. Far from abandoning the ill person or being selfish or evil, family members who are able to balance their lives between caretaking and autonomy are adapting in a healthy way. Helping in appropriate ways does not mean giving up one's own life entirely. This type of coping often helps to keep families intact, and actually strengthens the relationships between the various members.

Hugo and Rachel

◆ Despite his multiple sclerosis, Hugo and Rachel had been proud of the fact that they had reordered their lives and coped. He had been ill for several years, but with careful planning, the couple had been able to carry on a reasonably normal life, and had managed financially. All that changed, however, when Hugo's parents visited from Florida, and for the first time realized the extent of his disability. Without forewarning, they moved to the town Hugo and Rachel lived in, and began visiting frequently. Rachel had always had some difficulties with Hugo's mother because of her tendency to want to interfere in their affairs, but this was manageable as long as his parents lived in Florida. Now it became intolerable. Rachel was not spending enough time looking after Hugo; she should prepare extra meals for him on the weekends so that he would not have to prepare his own while she was at work; they should accept financial help from the parents so the house could be revamped to better handle his disability. The inadequacies—which previously had been inapparent to Rachel and Hugo—went on and on. Hugo did not want to hurt his parents' feelings, so he was reluctant to say anything to them; Rachel felt that if he did not do something soon, she would explode and so would their marriage. Before Hugo's parents arrived, she had felt that she was coping very well with their problems; now she felt exhausted all the time.

How members of the family handle a serious debilitating illness of a loved one has a great deal to do with how they personally react to illness. One way people react to illness, and the feelings of fear and guilt at seeing a child or family member ill, is by doing a great deal for them. Hugo's parents' overinvolvement with Hugo and criticism of Rachel may well represent their despair and panic about their son's illness. Their behavior is also a way to assert control over a situation which feels so out of control.

It is not uncommon for parents to express their fears and concerns by being critical of the child's spouse, in this case Rachel. When this happens, it tends to leave the spouse feeling not only inadequate, but also unsupported. It seems as if the only person who matters, who has feelings, needs, and problems, is the person with the physical illness. Spouses may feel a lack of support not only from the family but also from the medical community, because attention from the doctor is often directed solely toward the physical involvement, and not toward the impact of the illness on the family unit. This makes the wife or husband feel as if she/he must be very strong and never need help with the ill person or have any of her/his own needs met. A spouse put in this position may begin to feel anger, not only at in-laws (or other critical relatives) but also with the person suffering the medical condition for not supporting her/him against the accusations of the in-laws. Guilt, resentment, and the fear of making things worse for the ill person, can prevent the spouse from appropriately asserting herself/himself.

In this vignette, Rachel cannot wait for Hugo to recognize that his parents' involvement has created problems. She must tell Hugo how she feels, and perhaps they can plan a way to discuss things with her in-laws. This may be harder than it seems at first, because the ill person may like the extra attention he is getting by having his parents involved; this may result in his downplaying the detrimental effects of their intrusions. If this is the case, outside counseling should be sought, for without objections from their child, the involvement of the in-laws is likely to continue in the same way. If appropriate limits are not set within the family as to what is acceptable in terms of the in-laws' contributions, Rachel will continue to feel disenfranchised.

One way to set limits is to have a family meeting. A family meeting including the in-laws (or whoever the helping relative might be), is essential in these cases to clarify what is the most appropriate input of each person in helping the immediate family best adapt to the illness or injury. Rachel could use the support of her in-laws, but she cannot appreciate their help if she feels criticized and chastised. Hugo's parents want to be helpful, and could be utilized to decrease the burden on both Hugo and Rachel. It is important for them to provide support to the family, and very important for both Rachel and Hugo to have the help and comfort of the extended family. What seems to be missing is a constructive plan for how this can be accomplished.

At the family meeting, Rachel and Hugo can each explain what they see as the current needs they have, and what they think their future needs might be if the multiple sclerosis should worsen. They need to articulate what help they need now from Hugo's parents, and what help they anticipate they will need in the future. Hugo's parents can be called upon at this meeting to help generate ideas, and help make decisions about where Hugo and Rachel should live if they need to think about moving. They could be utilized to find out about some financial issues such as Social Security or disability benefits. If money is going to be a problem in the future, Hugo's parents might help in problem solving.

They can also be asked to do specific tasks. Hugo's mother could be asked to prepare some extra meals which could go into the freezer, for example. She and his father could go on some errands during the day, which Hugo would be unable to manage. Most importantly, Hugo needs to say something to his parents to help manage their behavior. For example, he could say, "Mom, Dad, I know you are anxious to help us and are worried about me. I am also worried and I appreciate your caring. However, it is very hard on Rachel and me if you are always making suggestions of how things could be done better. Let's sit down together and decide exactly what we need to have done and who is going to do what. We both want your help, but it has to be more organized. Also, I don't need you to visit every day. I want you to have a life of your own also. Please do that for me. Rachel also wants to have some time alone with me and to be able to invite you for dinner some time like normal people do. Let's work together to do this. OK?"

Any version of this can work. Often parents do not even realize how they have been interfering in the family rather than helping. It is easier than you might think to put into words what you are feeling and thinking. However family members will miss the point if you are angry, and if you sound like you are criticizing them. You can say what you want without getting others defensive, if you always preface it with a recognition of what the person(s) are trying to do for you and an appreciation of their efforts. Then feelings are not hurt, and the listener understands. Of course, this may not always be true. Regrettably, personalities are such that when a discussion like the foregoing occurs, the persons to whom it is directed will feel affronted. This is unfortunate, but it is necessary for the suffering family to maintain its integrity, and to do that, outside destructive forces must be addressed. Even when parents or others feel offended or unappreciated, these feelings are usually temporary and soon forgotten.

Finally, in some communities, the American Red Cross runs a multiple sclerosis course. (Other organizations devoted to other illnesses do similar things. A telephone call is all that it takes to find out what is available.) This course teaches families how to care for family members with multiple sclerosis. In Hugo and Rachel's case, it might be helpful to them if they suggested to Hugo's parents that they take the course. Rachel could go with them as well and this might give the three of them an opportunity to share their feelings and resolve their differences.

◆ Emotional exhaustion can come from a well partner taking on the entire burden, or from bending to unreasonable demands of the ill or disabled.

◆ Make sure that concerns about being seen as a good wife,

mother, child, do not result in unnecessary work, and the refusal of help.

♦ It is easy to underestimate what the ill or disabled person can do for him/herself and how he/she can help in the house. Be aware of this, so that the caretaker does not do more than is necessary.

♦ Get household help before the disease progresses.

♦ When managing a child's illness, keep things as normal as possible. Well siblings need opportunities to talk also.

♦ Teach children and all caretakers how to manage the illness calmly and responsibly.

♦ It is easy to become preoccupied with the sick child. Parents might work out a system where each parent checks the other to make sure that they are spending time with each child and not neglecting, overusing, or taking the well children for granted.

♦ Parents should not give up things in their lives for illness in a child, unless it is truly medically necessary.

♦ Even if the ill or disabled person expects you to provide all the care, that is not reasonable. It is important for you to resume appropriate goals and plans, so that you do not become emotionally exhausted.

CHAPTER 11

Handling Those Who Want to Help

Dealing with persons who either want to help in the event of chronic illness—or with those whose help might be welcomed, but who do not offer it—can be extremely stressful to the afflicted family. On the one hand, the help may be stifling and create increased tension in an already charged atmosphere; on the other hand, in many families, a bit of well-placed assistance might greatly ease the physical and emotional workload on the family members.

This chapter will offer suggestions in dealing with either of these situations. The first case is that of Julie who suffers sudden and severe disability, paralysis from the waist down, which does not worsen with time, but which does not improve either. This would be equally applicable to any person who has a stable but significant physical disability.

The second case is that of a young man (Jerry) who develops multiple sclerosis and has a progressively worsening course; again, a situation that might apply to any progressively debilitating and unpredictable illness. And the third case is that of a widow, Sadie, who has returned to work following her husband's death, and subsequently develops arthritis. This is an example of a disease which has a waxing and waning course, but which over-all becomes slowly worse. In each case, problems arise either because outside, well-meaning help was misplaced or necessary assistance was not forthcoming. Similar situations could occur in your family.

Julie

◆ Julie is a twenty-three-year-old model who was paralyzed from the waist down in a car accident. Her boyfriend of six months was soon gone, unable to cope with her permanent disability. His leaving coincided with Julie's imminent discharge from the hospital; so, instead of being able to return to the apartment they had shared, Julie had to go home to live with her mother. Julie's mother welcomed this idea because she felt that she understood her daughter better than anyone else, and could give her the best care. In the beginning, Julie appreciated the attention, but soon she began to wish her mother would let her comb her own hair, take her own baths, and in fact, manage most of her own hygiene. With a little time, Julie felt she might even be able to cook for herself. However, since she did not want to appear ungrateful, Julie did not say anything to her mother, but she spent more and more hours in her room watching TV and reading. Her mother felt very hurt by Julie's withdrawal and wondered if she was doing something wrong.

Parents, who naturally want to protect and care for their children, are very susceptible to feelings of overprotectiveness. If the parent is alone, as in Julie's case, offering help can quell feelings of helplessness, loneliness, and satisfy a wish to feel needed.

While assistance in the transition back to a fulfilling life-style may be indispensable, a disabled or ill person can become trapped in an invalid role, and recovery actually hampered. If everything is done for him, the disabled or ill person begins to believe that he is different, incompetent, and not a fully functioning person. Unfortunately, if someone like a parent, who early in the person's life took care of all his needs, reassumes and maintains that role in the face of medical crisis, the person loses independence and again feels infantilized. Despair and withdrawal are common reactions when an ill or disabled person realizes his position.

In fact, just the opposite kind of attitude needs to be encouraged. The person affected needs to begin to feel good about his changed or changing body, and he needs to re-establish a positive body image. If Julie does not take care of her own hygiene needs and grooming eventually, for example, she will avoid learning about her body and will not regain a sense of control. To prevent the potential trap of being overprotected by a parent or some other family member, and thus delaying the return of the ill or disabled person to a more independent life-style, limits must be set. Family members need to discuss with the ill or disabled person what they will do, and what the person will be expected to do. The disabled or ill person needs to make clear what is helpful, and what is not necessary because he/she is capable of doing it alone. If the person is going to live with a relative but hopes eventually to live on his/her own, then it is useful before moving in to set a time limit for how long the stay with that relative will be. This allows the ill or disabled person to set finite goals for re-establishing independence.

To achieve this sort of limit setting and planning, family members and the ill or disabled person have to make a conscious effort to sit down together and discuss all aspects of the posthospital plans, ideally before discharge. Once the plans have been made, all parties should make every attempt to stick to them. Sometimes it is helpful to do this with a professional who may have a more realistic appreciation of the situation, and thus is in an excellent position to give advice and concrete suggestions. If it is unclear exactly what a person can or cannot do for him/herself, physicians or nurses familiar with the person can participate in the planning. The disabled or ill person should have the last word; whatever he/she feels is right needs to be respected. Although having this type of family conference may at first seem difficult, it will ultimately avoid the misconceptions, hurt feelings, and confusion that are inevitable down the road without careful planning. If this type of planning did not occur at discharge, it is never too late to sit down with family and begin planning the best way to continue living and being together. Many families instinctively and naturally respond to the opinions and needs of the ill or disabled. But if this is not happening, it can be corrected through a family meeting and discussions.

◆ After living at home for six months, Julie felt able to try living in her own apartment. When she told her mother about this decision, her mother at first expressed approval and offered to help her find a suitable flat; but each time Julie suggested they go out apartment hunting, her mother was busy doing something else.

A parent, grandparent, or sibling may become very involved in caring for a child, even an adult child, and may like the feeling of being needed and having the companionship of the ill or disabled person. The parent may be trying to in some way make up for the devastation of the injury (illness), and in so doing may be able to resolve his/her own feelings of anger over what has happened, or resolve vague guilt that he/she ought to have prevented it from happening. This can prevent adaptive and healthy adjustment to one's forever-changed life. If this is happening, as in Julie's case, either Julie or another family member may have to gently confront the parent. Again, it may be easier for a social worker, chaplain, or other counselor to speak with the parent in such a circumstance. Short-term family therapy can be helpful to get families through this critical decision-making phase of adjustment.

◆ Julie was eventually able to find a suitable apartment. At first all went well, and Julie began to feel very confident of her ability to take care of herself. She was ecstatic when offered a job counseling young models at her old agency. Back at work, however, she soon found that managing all her household tasks, cooking, and cleaning was taking more time than she had. Her mother offered to come and help out, but Julie was hesitant.

Julie is understandably uncertain about her mother's reentry into her new life. She has good reason to be wary that Mom may again try to take over. At times, however, even with a previously unsettling experience, outside help can be acceptable from a parent or other family member. However, it is vital that before the help is accepted, appropriate limits be set so that the family members can contribute in constructive ways. And the person or family receiving the help must resolve to terminate it if the bounds are overstepped. Julie needs to tell her mother exactly what help she wants from her. If her mother cannot do only what she has been asked to do, and intrudes into other areas of her life, then other alternatives will have to be pursued. Julie cannot blame her mother if Julie has not been clear and laid down the rules ahead of time. This frequently happens and is as much the fault of the ill or disabled person as it is of the caretaker. It would be unfortunate if Julie could not use her mother's help if she wanted to. It may be the best alternative available to her. If not too intrusive, Julie's mother's assistance could provide both of them with support and help.

An ill or disabled person may not recognize or realize until living alone what his/her capacity is for taking care of home and work. This is a problem that all of us who face a full day of work and then household duties also must cope with, but the dimensions are magnified for those with chronic illness or disability. There is no need to prove that one is super human to establish one's personal independence. Hiring a housekeeper to help with shopping and cleaning needs is often a wise decision for anyone.

When help is hired, one should make clear what the responsibilities of that person are. If there are special needs as a result of an illness or disability, this ought to be made clear before the person is hired. If finances are a problem, government funds may be available for assistance, or family members may offer financial help. But, again in this area, appropriate limits must be set ahead of time. It may seem difficult to sit down with family members and set limits on financial or any other type of assistance. But it is much easier to do this than to try to pick up the pieces after a major family fight erupts because of resentments caused when someone, likely well meaning, intrudes into the afflicted person's "space."

An alternative approach is to team up with another person with similar problems. Two spinal-cord disabled persons or two persons with cerebral palsy can often live together and help each other out. While this kind of arrangement can be very satisfying both economically and socially, issues of privacy are important, and again rules and limits will need to be worked out ahead of time.

Jerry and Pam

◆ Multiple sclerosis did not seem like such a bad disease five years ago when Jerry first heard the diagnosis. At that time he had lost the feeling in his left leg for two days, but it had returned. However, the term *MS* had become much more ominous in the last six months, since he had been experiencing increasing difficulty with coordination and walking. During this time, his wife Pam had been finding her life much changed and was having problems coping. She had gotten their son Andrew off to school in the morning and then concentrated on April, her two-year-old daughter. Now she was needed to help get Jerry dressed and had to drive him to work. It was like having a new baby! By noon she was exhausted. The young couple had been quite outgoing and usually spent one night a week entertaining, or enjoying movies and theater. But with Jerry's increasing debility, both were too tired to even want social activities.

Jerry's mother, with whom he was very close, offered to come in the mornings and help get Jerry dressed and ready for work. At first this seemed like a godsend to Pam, but soon she had the feeling that she was no longer needed by her husband; Jerry and his mother seemed to rely totally on each other, and any suggestions or requests Pam made were either ignored or criticized. Pam began to feel uncomfortable around her own husband.

Jerry's mother was shocked to learn the depths of her daughter-in-law's frustration. She had been so involved in the care of her oldest son and so anguished over his illness, that she had completely ignored the rest of the family. She had been so concentrated on her son that she had forgotten the birthday of her grandchild April, whom she cherished. One day April said to her, "Nana, if my head aches like Daddy's, would you rub it for me?" It had been months since she and April had enjoyed an afternoon together, a treat both she and April had previously enjoyed every Friday.

Over-involvement in the care of an ill person can sneak up on even the most well-meaning person! The constant questioning and balancing act is, "How much is enough but not too much?" It is important for anyone helping in this way to step back every once in a while and take a look at the situation to insure that his/her involvement is not interfering in the primary family relationships of both the sick person and him/herself. Because the needs of a chronically ill person can seem overwhelming at times, it is sometimes difficult to step back, but this is necessary for the benefit of everyone.

In the example of Jerry's family, not only his wife and daughter, but his mother as well were hurt by her well-intended but overly focused care. In a family with chronic illness, the non-ill members need the support and appreciation of in-laws and others with whom they are close; when attention becomes concentrated on the ill person, these people suffer from emotional neglect. In young families, the loss is double for the children, because the mother or father is often less available because of the new demands—almost like that of a new child—placed on her/him. If other close relatives, like grandparents, can maintain or enhance their relationships with their grandchildren in these circumstances, it can make it much easier for the parents to meet the children's emotional needs without becoming exhausted. Often this kind of help is the best kind of help relatives can offer. It also allows the well member of the family to feel less guilty about time spent caring for the sick person.

A second family unit at risk of being neglected is that of the well-meaning relative. That person can become so involved in the ill person's care that his/her spouse or children are left to fend for themselves. This can result in angry feelings and ultimately a breakdown of previously good relationships if the problem is either not recognized, or if recognized, not acted upon. As in most such situations, maintaining good communication with all the involved parties often prevents crisis. If the participation of the person offering help is resented by his/her spouse, but is truly needed by the family suffering chronic illness, it is sometimes possible to include the resentful spouse in the care. For example, both grandparents can do things together with grandchildren, offering them much-needed attention and security. How the joint input of grandparents, for example, can be accommodated, will vary from family to family and must be tailored to each family's particular needs.

◆ Unfortunately, Jerry's mother was unable to distance herself from Jerry's immediate care. Pam found herself very resentful of what now seemed to be interference in her private life and the life of her family. Still she found it difficult to tell her mother-in-law that she no longer wanted her help. In the course of a few months, as Pam became increasingly angry at her mother-in-law, her anger shifted over to her husband. She became irritable, distant, and one day approached him with the suggestion that he move back in with his parents.

The increasing demands and stress of a progressive illness on family members can lead to emotional exhaustion (see also Chapter 10: Preventing Emotional Exhaustion, Hugo and Rachel), resentment, and disillusionment. The well partner in the family needs non-illness–related time with the ill person; it is very easy to slip into spending one's time to the point of exhaustion filling all the needs related to that 'third person', the illness, and neglect the primary relationship with the person. It may seem as if there just are not enough hours in the day to meet the demands of the illness and still maintain a loving relationship, and give the kids the attention they need.

You need to make time! Now is the time to call in that well-meaning relative, and redirect his/her involvement in the family. Thank the person for the help he/she has given. However, tell them that you have noticed that you and your spouse are starting to grow apart, and now you need them to take on a different and more important task. You need the relative to get the kids out of the house and allow you and your spouse to spend some time together alone. You have decided that you are going to hire some household help as well. In this or a similar way, the help of outsiders can often be directed into truly beneficial avenues. To remain in control of your household and your life, you must tell your helpers—yes, you have a *right* to do this—exactly what they can do that will be helpful. This will prevent them from deciding for themselves where their input should be.

Unfortunately, alas, even when the most diplomatic means are used to redirect or refuse such help, the person involved can become angry or upset, and feel that the family is ungrateful. However, it is important to remember that the feelings of the outsider are *not* more important than the integrity of the family unit suffering the illness. Sometimes anger and bad feelings cannot be avoided; if they are necessary to keep the family from disintegrating, then that is the way it must be. In time, such feelings can be resolved; once the rules of the family interrelationships have been established and limits set, everyone involved ultimately feels better.

Sadie

◆ Sadie was widowed at age sixty when her husband died of a heart attack. After a few months, she resumed her twenty-year-long career as a sales supervisor in a large department store. Besides her job, Sadie had been actively involved in a local gardening club and in her church. Then, at age sixty-two, she began to experience pain and stiffness in her finger and knee joints. Initially she called it old-age arthritis, but when it continued and did not respond to simple painkillers, she visited her family doctor. He told her that she had rheumatoid arthritis. She would need to reorder her life. More rest, more medication, and special exercises were to be a part of her life from now on.

Sadie tried to adhere to all the instructions; nevertheless the pain and stiffness lasted longer in the mornings; at times she could hardly walk. Her fingers became more swollen, and she had trouble holding things and opening them. She was forced to drop to half-time at work; then her employer offered her early retirement. Though she felt very frustrated, Sadie had always been very independent and fought to continue on her own. She hid her illness from her family. Late one morning, Carl, Sadie's thirty-year-old son, dropped in unexpectedly. He was shocked to find not only that she was just getting up but also what a difficult time she was having just walking around the house, obviously in pain.

Two weeks later, Carol, Sadie's daughter, invited her for a family dinner. When Sadie arrived, Carol and Carl led her into the living room where the coffee table was spread with brochures on different condominiums. "We think you should be moving nearer to us," Carol began. Sadie did not know what to do. She listened politely as her children went through the various advertisements. She heard nothing of what they said. She could hardly wait to get to her own home.

Children, even adult children, can be quite alarmed when they first realize the vulnerabilities of their aging parents. They have an immediate desire to rush in and help the parent. Sometimes unintentionally, they can take actions that they feel are appropriate; but without the parent's knowledge, it is inappropriate. Rather than helping the parent, this unexpected intrusion on his/her life can be very frightening and confusing.

After living in a community for many years, people feel very secure and oriented. They know the shopkeepers in the neighborhood and the community figures, and have long-standing friends— they belong. The home they live in is filled with memories and is both comforting and comfortable. To be wrested out of this environment, especially for an elderly person or a person who has recently lost a loved one, can cause extreme anxiety, disorientation, and depression. New communities, even for young people, can be cold and isolating until new friends can be found. This process is much prolonged, if it can be accomplished, by an older person who can no longer work and who has a disabling illness. It is impossible for children to decide what is best for an ailing parent, without consulting with the parent if that person is mentally competent. What is most convenient for the children may in fact result in the loss of independence and impaired quality of life for the parent.

This is another example in which well-meaning help can be disastrous, if the feelings and input of all persons affected are not considered before action is taken. In Sadie's case, remaining in her familiar community is very important if she can possibly manage it. Often, a relatively simple solution can be worked out if the parties to the problem can sit down and talk about it. Carol and Carl, after discussing the options with Sadie, agreed to contribute toward hiring a part-time housekeeper who could do grocery shopping and laundry. This allowed Sadie to maintain her independence and her social activities with her old friends.

◆ Though everyone had agreed, and it had been decided that Sadie would stay in her own home, Carl was concerned. Twice a week, he would drop by to make sure everything was all right. However, this drive added an extra hour commuting time, and he realized that he would soon have to drop out of his racquetball club. Why couldn't his mother move nearer so that these problems could be avoided? Sadie, for her part, could feel the tension developing in her relationship with Carl. While she loved seeing him, she began to feel anxiety before his visits and wished she did not have to impose on him. She began to wonder if it would not have been easier to move to one of those condominiums.

The relationships of children and parents are very complex. Feelings of obligation, and fear of losing independence coexist with the love and sincere desire to make the parent's later years as enjoyable as possible. The conflict of these feelings, and the attempts of the child to act appropriately on them and yet maintain an independent life, can be difficult.

In this case, enough stresses were being created and not diffused by communication between the two parties, that their relationship was threatened by tension and resentment. Of course, the ideal situation is to be able to sit down and talk about the feelings of the persons involved when a relationship begins to crack, but this is not always possible, especially between parents and grown children. The child's sense of obligation, especially to a parent who wishes to maintain an independent life-style, is not necessarily shared by the parent. That is, Sadie likely would prefer that her son visit when convenient; not because he feels it is necessary. She does not feel it is necessary.

Carl's feeling that he is the one who must make sure Mom is OK may be a reflection of how he perceives his role in the family, or what he considers is expected of him as the only son. However, these visits are clearly interfering with his life-style; and for her part, Sadie would just as soon her needs not be met out of a sense of obligation. To her, it is not important that her son be the only one that helps her; what is important is that the tasks get done. A housekeeper, part-time gardener, and local grocery that will deliver, will fill her needs. Often, for other less frequent tasks, like shoveling snow, carrying things in from the car, etc., neighbors' teenagers or preteens will be more than willing to make some money. Sometimes a neighbor would help with jobs like gardening or shoveling snow. Community services, such as Meals on Wheels and visiting nurse associations, offer specialized services. Visiting nurses can provide Sadie with physical therapy, as well as share knowledge about services in the community. In appropriate situations, devices are available—like jar-opening aids—to patients with particular disabilities (see Chapter 5: Finding and Using Community Resources), and many associations dealing with specific illnesses will assist sufferers in obtaining these. Local chapter phone numbers can usually be gotten right out of the white pages. The Arthritis Foundation (see Appendix 1) offers educational programs, such as the Arthritis Self-Help Course and Joint Efforts Exercise Program, which is taught by a physical therapist to help people with arthritis learn exercises to help reduce their pain.

With the onus of expectations removed from the child's mind, he/she can visit the parent, because he/she wants to, and will be able to maintain a more normal relationship that both can enjoy. At the same time, the child's life-style need not be disrupted.

◆ Sadie hired a neighbor and a local teenager to help her with tasks around the house, and things with Carl went much better. Still, her disease kept her confined to the house most of the time. She had always been fastidious about her appearance and regularly had her hair dyed and shaped at a nearby salon. Recently, however, the two-hour sitting, plus the trip back and forth, had become exhausting. Her daughter was a beauty operator, and Sadie often wished that she could ask Carol if she would mind doing her hair once a month. Because of the way things had turned out with Carl, though, Sadie did not know what to do. She did not want to be a burden to her daughter too.

This is a perfect example of a way in which a child could be of indispensable assistance to an ailing parent, and it would not be a burden. Sadie's need for a service her daughter is uniquely equipped to provide occurs at most once a month. Likely, a child would be most willing to provide this sort of help and may even be flattered that the parent would ask for it.

While adult children should not be expected to always be available for a parent, there is also a danger in being too independent. It is alright for a parent to ask for help, especially when he/she is becoming too isolated because of fears of becoming a burden. It is important for each family to learn to distinguish at what point in their interrelationships the involvement moves from mutually beneficial to interference. Carl's twice-weekly visits were destructive in this case; however, Carol's monthly help with Sadie's hair and perhaps bimonthly lunch and shopping dates, could be mutually enjoyed. What is right or best will vary from family to family as well, as with the degree of debility of the ill person. What is critical is that all family members be attuned to each other's needs and feelings, and make the effort to come up with alternatives that do not burden anyone.

◆ Parents of adult children may experience a very strong need to protect and care for that child if he/she becomes seriously injured or ill. While help is often necessary and appreciated, definite limits should be imposed so that the child is allowed to remain independent, and the help does not become interference.

◆ When relatives become involved in helping out, they must be careful to preserve their own relationships. If a parent or sibling feels needed by a sick family member, it is easy to neglect his/her spouse, children, or grandchildren. The result can be increased suffering and division in the family.

◆ Relatives may be called upon to do specific, defined tasks which will allow the family members a bit of free time. Such tasks might include, e.g., baby-sitting children, sitting with the ill person for a few hours, or driving him/her to a medical appointment.

◆ Adult children are often called upon to help ailing parents. These responsibilities should be shared among siblings. While children should be available to help parents, they must be careful to strike a balance so as not to neglect their own families.

◆ All help need not come from family or friends. Community services should be accessed whenever possible to lessen the load of afflicted families.

CHAPTER 12

Maintaining Intimacy

The intimate ties between two people are difficult to maintain under the best of circumstances. Relationships even among well people will falter, if the people involved do not constantly work to keep the relationship alive and healthy.

When illness, or physical or mental disability, becomes a part of a couple's life, everything becomes more complex. It is almost as if three people are living together—the two partners and the medical problem. This intruder invariably disrupts the old relationship, and the new feelings it evokes need to be recognized and dealt with before the partners can be intimate again. In many ways the couple may have to start all over—almost as if they were dating again. To renew intimacy at a sexual level, partners must feel comfortable with each other and feel good about being together. This rarely "just happens"; it requires time and communication.

In the vignettes in this chapter, we talk about some of the common reactions to illness or disability that interfere with a couple's ability to maintain an intimate relationship. We offer ways to reestablish feelings of intimacy. Two of the couples, Helen and Robert (diabetes mellitus), and George and Marie (heart attack), are middle to late middle-age and have been married for some time. Their intimate relationships have been disrupted by medical illnesses. Mike and Kim are a young couple trying to cope with the effects of spinal-cord injury, and Lisa is a young single woman with a disfiguring bowel operation, who is trying to reestablish close relationships after having lost one because of the surgery.

Helen and Robert

◆ Helen and Robert had been married thirty years. Each had a successful career; he as a lawyer, and she as an executive. They had two grown sons with whom they were very close. About twenty years ago, Robert had developed diabetes mellitus, which was a common disease in his family. Though he had had to take insulin injections for a number of years, this had not had a major impact on his life, and he felt fortunate he had had no complications from his illness. Over the last several months, though, he noticed that he was having more and more difficulty getting and maintaining an erection. This bothered him. He wondered if he were just getting old, or if he were losing his desire for Helen. He found himself thinking about this problem a lot, and found more and more excuses to avoid sexual encounters with his wife.

Frequently, men with diabetes mellitus will experience erection problems and/or low sexual desire. Often a combination of emotional and physical factors result in the sexual dysfunctioning. Normal changes in sexual functioning attributable to aging, such as a lengthening in the time it takes to get an erection, or the need for more caressing by a partner to achieve an erection, as well as changes in the orgasm, frequently occur in diabetic men at a younger age than in men who do not have diabetes mellitus. If the man with diabetes has not been educated about these changes, they may cause undue concern and panic. Specific suggestions about sexuality and diabetes can be found in *Sexuality and Chronic Illness,* by Schover and Jensen. (See Appendix 2.)

Often, as in Robert's case, the inability to achieve an erection or the loss of an erection is perceived by the man as a real blow to his virility and sense of masculinity, especially if he is already suffering from a chronic illness. He will likely not attribute these changes to the illness or to complications of the illness unless he has been forewarned that they might occur. Fears will almost inevitably develop about his future ability to be a lover and partner capable of providing sexual satisfaction, and receiving the same in return. The additional stress this causes, and Robert is a good example, then may result in the loss of sexual desire. The vicious cycle is completed, and the person's intimate relationship(s) will undoubtedly suffer or dissolve. Thoughts of waning or unpredictable sexual ability and loss of masculinity also cause fear and embarrassment. It is important to remember that these feelings are a common response to changes in one's body and health as a result of the illness. Feelings of depression, unattractiveness, or anxiety about the future can affect sexual desire and performance as well. With all of these assaults to one's self-image that accompany chronic illnesses, it becomes easy to find excuses for not having sex.

◆ Before Robert told Helen about his impotence, she had been very worried. She had noticed that Robert was less interested in having sex with her and began to wonder if he were having an affair. She began to feel hurt and jealous, and found herself arguing with him over minor issues.

When one sexual partner withdraws from a relationship, the other often misses the closeness of their long sexual contact. In this case, Helen feels rejected and sexually unattractive, and does not even consider the possibility that her partner's illness, or the impact of the illness, might be involved. When there are no outward physical changes from illness, it is common to forget that there are potential complications that may affect other members of the family. It seems that Helen was unaware that diabetes might be at fault, and she imagined all sorts of things that caused her pain and stress. Her stress could have been lessened if she could have asked her husband why he was acting so differently toward her. Robert's feelings of embarrassment and fear, as well as Helen's feelings of rejection, may leave little time for them to think about each other. If they can talk about their fears, they can reassure each other that they are sexually attractive and desirable. They may both be surprised to learn that although they miss intercourse, they have also been as concerned about the loss of holding, touching, and closeness. Robert may be able to confide his fears about his losses. Frequently, changes in sexual functioning arise as an illness progresses, and result in a couple having to learn to readjust and cope with new insults of an illness to which they thought they had adjusted. Just to be faced with the fact that a disease is progressing can be discouraging, and add stress to the couple's attempts to cope with a changing sexual relationship.

◆ When it had been explained to the couple that Robert's problem probably was a result of his illness, they were able to once again establish good communication. They developed a new closeness through kissing, touching, and holding. However, both felt that something was missing; it was not the same as when they were able to satisfy each other through sexual intercourse.

It may not be the same, but it can be very enjoyable. Many couples feel they have lost something they had together, and they may each feel angry and sad about it. It is normal to feel anger and grief over such a loss. At this time, a couple needs to talk about what, short of intercourse, feels sexually satisfying to each of them. Closeness comes from sharing feelings and providing what each person needs to feel satisfied sexually. Sexual devices, films, vacations together, candlelight dinners, showers, mutual massages, or mutual masturbation, all bring a closeness and sexual sharing that may be more intimate than intercourse. Sexual sharing does not depend on any one technique. There is no right way or one way that guarantees satisfaction. The focus on intercourse and orgasm frequently takes away from a focus on enjoying each other, and enjoying lovemaking. However, if intercourse is very important, penile implants can be considered. Penile implants are devices that can surgically be permanently placed in the man's penis and used to create an artificial erection, so that the man can penetrate the vagina. This alternative can allow continued sexual intercourse. Each couple needs to make their own decision whether this is their best route to mutual sexual satisfaction. It is important also that a medical examination by a urologist be done to determine whether or not physical damage from diabetes, or other illness or injury, is the cause of the erectile problems. If this is the case, rather than primarily emotional or stress factors, then a penile implant may be a viable alternative. Decisions about the use of prosthesis (an implant) might be better made in consultation with a urologist, sex therapist, or counselor, but it certainly becomes an option. Whether or not physical damage or emotional issues alone are involved, the couple may need to focus on new ways to enjoy each other sexually as the result of chronic illness. This is particularly true, since the medical problems will almost certainly affect many other aspects of their life, and may affect the ill person's ability to move (e.g., arthritis), or his/her physical appearance. Through the process of counseling, couples can receive information about the diversity of sexuality and sexual satisfaction, and an awareness of how restrictive beliefs (if we can't have sexual intercourse, then it is no good) can prevent sexual satisfaction.

George and Marie

◆ George would never forget the day he had his heart attack. He was in his prime—a hard-driving, respected accountant who had become a major partner in a large firm. On that day, he was presenting to a new client, when a crushing pain in his chest made him gasp for breath. The next thing he remembered was waking up in intensive care and seeing his wife, Marie, standing over his bed with tears in her eyes. Within a few days he learned he had sustained serious heart damage and nearly died. He was only fifty-two!

After his early recuperation, he was sent home on special diet, several medications, and a graded exercise program. George found himself obsessed with the feeling that he was going to have another heart attack. He limited his activities to sitting in front of the television and eating. One of the activities his physician told him he could resume, but which he had not, was sex. He was terribly frightened that intercourse would cause another heart attack. Everytime he had an erection, these fears would surface, and he would lose it.

Often, heart-attack survivors like George are afraid that it is not safe to resume sexual activity. They are preoccupied with themselves and their mortality; their self-esteem and self-image have been dealt a crushing blow. The fear of sudden death, and the dread of going back into a hospital, can be overwhelming, and can deprive them of the satisfaction of returning to a normal life that includes recreational activities and work-related activities, as well as sexual activities.

Fears about worsening one's medical condition or dying during sexual activity are common. The medical doctor should be asked whether there is any particular risk from sexual activity, or in the case of a particular event like a heart attack or a recent surgery, when it is safe to resume a normal sex life. It is important to ask the doctor these questions about your sex life, because the answer varies from individual to individual even with the same condition, depending on the severity of the condition, the level of activity that person has returned to, and his personal life-style (exercise, drinking, smoking, and diet). The ill person's sexual partner may have fears about harming the person or killing him/her during sex as well and should be included in any discussions. The couple need to let each other know about their fears and talk about their fear of dying.

In discussing the resumption of sexual activity, it is also important to find out if any of the new medications you may have been placed on affect sexual function. Some medications, especially some of those used to treat high blood pressure and coronary artery disease, can affect sexual performance by causing problems in reaching an erection for some men.

Once these issues are discussed and the necessary changes in medication are made, and necessary changes in sexual activity— if any, and many times there are none—have been discussed, then good communciation between the person with the illness or disability and the partner is essential for the resumption of sexual activity. If position changes are necessary to control for shortness of breath or pain, for example, new positions can be discussed and practiced. If a female partner is upset about being more active or getting on top, traditionally a male role, this attitude needs to be discussed, and she can be reassured that this is acceptable and enjoyable to her spouse. Understanding that negative attitudes about women being active and sexual may come from a misunderstanding of the cultural and family conditioning a woman gets when growing up, makes it seem more likely that these negative attitudes can be overcome. These discussions can help begin a process of re-education. Husbands, wives, or lovers often begin this education process as the result of an illness that requires changes in sexual behavior.

Sometimes sexual devices such as a vibrator or sex films can be used to increase excitement and shorten the length of time to complete the sex act. Use of a dildo or penis stiffener can enable sexual intercourse when it might not be possible otherwise. A dildo is a semi-hard rubber, artificial penis which can be used by hand or by strapping it to the penis. Use of a dildo gives the experience of vaginal penetration. A stiffener is made of hard rubber and fits over the penis, keeping it stiff enough for intercourse. Persons who may have fairly rigid feelings about sex or many religious or other inhibitions regarding sex, may feel uncomfortable, fearful, and concerned about the changes. If this type of feeling exists, it needs to be brought up and discussed, and if it cannot be resolved, the couple may benefit from professional sexual counseling.

A couple who is communicating well might mutually agree through discussion that just hugging and kissing can be satisfying, and that every time intimacy is shared it does not have to lead to intercourse. This realization can be a great relief to the ill person, and can remove the partner's fears of hurting the ill person's feelings. It can also remove guilt in both parties about being satisfied with less. The need for increased stimulation, as well as other preferences to improve sexual functioning, are now exceedingly important to communicate. It is often beneficial to seek outside sex counseling to learn how to communicate, learn ways to engage in safe sexual activities, and to prevent more serious marital conflict and depression. If avoidance of sexual activity after a serious illness is also serving to end what was an unsatisfying sexual life before the onset of the injury or illness, counseling may be an opportunity to resolve past difficulties, and begin enjoying a renewed sexual relationship.

◆ Marie had been present when the doctor talked about George's resuming a sexual relationship. However, six months had passed since the heart attack, and though sex had been mentioned several times, George had always claimed he was too tired or weak. Meanwhile, Marie was having dreams about sexual encounters and found herself attracted to one of her coworkers. She was becoming more and more concerned about her appearance and realized she was considering an affair. As soon as she had these thoughts, she felt ashamed. They were both devout Catholics, and she knew he would not do something like this. Besides, it was a sin.

When a sexually active woman experiences a long and unexpected hiatus in a previously fulfilling relationship, she may feel rejected and sexually undesirable. She may feel very hurt and angry at her partner for his apparent disinterest; at the same time she feels guilty about feeling this way, because after all, the partner cannot control the fact he is ill. Often a wife will not talk to her partner about these feelings for several reasons; she may feel guilty, or it may be hard to verbalize the feelings, or he may be difficult to talk to because of his preoccupation with himself.

It is common in this situation to fantasize about other men (or women if the woman is ill), who will not reject your sexual advances. An affair in this case is one way to experiment with other possibilities, and for a while to distance oneself from one's spouse and the difficulties of resolving the current sexual problems. Yet, these thoughts can bring added guilt especially if, like the couple here, religious beliefs play an important role in this aspect of their lives or they have strong beliefs about adultery.

Thoughts and feelings are not actions and do not constitute adultery; the well partner does not need to feel guilt and shame about fantasies, for they are very common experiences for sexually healthy people and are a healthy way of finding a sexual outlet.

Most importantly, Marie should share her feelings and fears. She might create a special setting in which to broach the subject. She might prepare a favorite meal and afterwards suggest that they talk about their sex life with the provision that all he needs to do is listen to her and not necessarily respond. This is not a time to blame each other but just to state how one is feeling. All sentences should start with the word "I." "I" statements are not accusatory. If Marie can state how she feels without asking George a question about how he feels, she can express what she is really feeling. A good exercise is to set aside ten minutes every night at a convenient time. Using a clock, each person speaks to the other for five minutes uninterruptedly. The nonspeaking spouse does not respond but only listens. After five minutes the speaker becomes the listener. No responses are necessary; it is only necessary to try to understand what each other is saying. Eventually this can lead to problem solving once the problems have been identified.

Mike and Kim

◆ Mike and Kim, a young couple in their twenties, were returning from a vacation in New England when a deer suddenly appeared in front of their car, causing Mike, who was driving, to swerve off the road and into a tree. Fortunately, their two-year-old son, who was in a car seat, was only bruised, but both Kim and Mike had serious injuries. Kim's broken arm and lacerations healed quickly, but it soon became apparent that Mike would remain paralyzed from a broken neck that left him with no leg function, and minimal arm and hand function.

In the first year after the accident, Kim and Mike's time was taken up with coping with Mike's disability, his rehabilitation, and Kim's need to find a job and a house that was suitable for Mike. Kim also needed to arrange child care for Eric, which before the accident was not necessary. Although Kim and Mike had had an active sex life prior to the accident, they had never really talked about sex and knew very little about each other's likes, dislikes, and needs. Since the accident, the couple had had no sex.

Mike and Kim are not unusual in that the quality of the sexual relationship is often one of the least discussed facets of a couple's life. Two partners may not even know the things that each other likes the most sexually. When one partner becomes ill or disabled, then the couple has no basis from which to initiate discussions about their future sex life; they usually feel uneasy discussing sexual issues. In the early stages of injury or illness, there always seems to be much more serious life-threatening issues to deal with. This allows a couple to justify putting off facing the inevitable sexual issues for long periods of time, although both may frequently think about their sexuality. These are inevitable issues, not only because of each person's inherent need for closeness and sex—whether sick or not—but also because in North American society and culture, one's sexuality is a major aspect of one's identity.

It is very helpful when there are sexuality education programs that are a part of the rehabilitation process. Hospital personnel— psychologists, social workers, nurses, or doctors—can assist a couple in initiating discussions about their new sexual relationship even before the ill or injured person goes home. Frequently, however, the lack of educational programs, hospital staffs' own discomfort with the subject, frequent negative attitudes by staff about the possibility of the resumption of sexual activities, and the failure to perceive that sexuality will be a major area of adjustment, prevents this from happening.

Therefore, it is not surprising that the couple in this vignette, or indeed the majority of couples facing similar situations, may go for months or even years without resuming any sexual relationship. Communication is essential. This is particularly difficult for the couple who has never talked about sex. Initiating discussions is a way of saying to one's partner, "Look, I know things are different now, but I still love you and want to have sex with you, so let's figure out how we can do it." It is a way of reassuring the ill or injured person that he/she is still attractive; an essential ingredient to resuming sexual activity. It is not uncommon for a man to find out during such a discussion, for example, that a woman does not actually mind foregoing intercourse, as she always preferred hugging, kissing, and touching anyway. Once he realizes this and knows that intercourse, of which he may be incapable, is not expected of him, he can consider that he could still approach his mate sexually and satisfy her needs. Men, as well as women, can experience considerable satisfaction and comfort from hugging and lying close together.

♦ Although Mike had had fantasies, he had not shared these experiences with Kim and felt that sex was over for him. While he did on occasion have an erection, the fact that he had no control over them and could not initiate sex made it all the more frustrating. This was such a private and embarrassing subject for him that he had not even talked about it with his doctors. Furthermore, he could hardly bear to look at his shriveling legs and protruding belly, which made him feel out of shape and old.

Mike's reactions are very common after injury. It is a devastating time for anyone suffering a major disabling illness or injury. The results of physical changes can be feelings of repulsiveness about one's body and a certainty that others are equally repulsed. This can make the person feel ugly and create a negative body image. The physical disability becomes stigmatizing. Self-esteem is very dependent at this time on one's partner's reactions and the reactions of other people to the disabled person. Feeling socially weird or strange does not increase self-esteem. Physical appearance plays a role in physical attractiveness and sexual arousal. Culturally in our society, good looks and youth have been associated with sexual attractiveness and desire. Most importantly, each person forms an opinion about his own attractiveness and sexual desirability, which dictates how comfortable he is in social interactions and how often he engages in social activities. Sexual self-esteem is highly related to each person's feelings about his/her physical self—the body and its physical attributes. Physical disabilities or chronic illnesses, such as multiple sclerosis or Parkinson's Disease, alter a person's physical appearance. Since, culturally, our society has had little tolerance for the *appearance* of disabilities, physical changes in mobility and distortions of features have cast labels on victims as "repulsive." Therefore, when people experience a disabling injury, such as spinal-cord injury, they may believe that they are sexually unattractive and undesirable. For many, including physicians and other health-care professionals, it is easy to feel that sexual activity must be over. Fears of rejection because of loss of sexual self-esteem can prevent single men or women from attempting to meet others, and from exposing themselves to situations in which they can socialize. These same feelings can lead married couples to withdraw sexually from each other. If friends and family members treat the ill or disabled person as if he/she is helpless and childlike, and not as independent, fully functioning adults, this sends a message that affects the injured person's sexual self-esteem. If one's partner initiates affection, touching, and hugging, it tells the injured or ill person that they are still sexually attractive.

Mike's preinjury attitudes and beliefs about his sexuality will play a role also. Unusually rigid attitudes about male sex roles and embarrassment about sexual activities would make it difficult for Mike to bring up his sexual concerns. Frequently when erections are sporadic or nonexistent, and when orgasm has been impaired, people feel sex must be over. Rigid and misinformed attitudes about who properly initiates sex, as well as rigid attitudes about the conduct of intercourse, can also lead to this conclusion. Of course, some of this rigidity may just reflect ignorance about the functioning of sexual organs, and what might constitute sexual satisfaction. For example, it is a common but erroneous belief that if there is no erection and intercourse, nothing is felt, or it is being done in a bad way. This belief certainly would eliminate alternative options that the couple might engage in. When a spouse is as uncomfortable as Mike is about talking about sex, it may be helpful for the able-bodied spouse to make the first overtures. Actions can speak louder than words. Hugs, touches, and kisses can help to send the message that Mike is desirable and desired. Through Kim's overtures, encouragement, and acknowledgment of her pleasure, Mike can learn how to satisfy her and himself. He may get considerable satisfaction, in fact, just out of being able to please her.

It can be helpful if spouses sit down before having any sexual activity, and begin discussing their attitudes and beliefs about sex. Each can take a turn telling the other all the thoughts and feelings they have about sex, which they have learned over the years. It can be very enlightening to hear what the other one really thinks. Then each person tells the other what is enjoyable about the sex act for them. There is no requirement to have sex, only to listen to each other and to be as honest as one can. This type of discussion often leads to changes in attitudes and choices of sexual activity in bed. It is wrong to assume that a man knows everything about sex because he is a man. Men and women need to learn about alternative ways to have sex, and about those things that stimulate a woman and man. Going to the library and taking out books on the subject is a good way to become educated.

It is very important to become educated about the physiologic fundamentals of the sex act after a disabling illness or injury. Sex is certainly not over. Changes have to take place. For example, often as a result of the losses of mobility, preferred positions are no longer possible or comfortable, certain bowel or bladder preparations have to be made, supportive pillows have to be arranged, and intercourse or sexual activities have to be timed to avoid pain or to catch erections. Catheters can be removed or positioned out of the way so that using a catheter or urine bag does not have to prevent sexual activity. If a bag cannot be removed because of an ileostomy for example, a drainage tube can be used to connect from the bag to a drainage bottle. There are many hints to learn so that urine-collection bags and tubes need not prevent sex. One can learn about these things from experimenting or from talking to others who are physically disabled who have handled these problems. Besides finding ways to use traditional positioning, experimenting with positions that are comfortable and work for each individual, depending on the limitations of the disability, can bring satisfaction. Sitting in and using the wheelchair, either in a bedroom or in a roll-in shower, or lying side-by-side rather than on top or under are alternatives not frequently considered by couples, but which can work very effectively.

Following such an injury or in the face of other disabling illnesses, a couple needs to spend some time exploring each other's bodies to find areas that enhance their sexual feelings. After spinal-cord injury, other areas of the body gain more sensitivity, such as the breasts and nipples; and touching of these areas can be very sexually arousing. Remaining lovers in some sense and doing so in part by ongoing discussion of their sexual relationship, will help to preserve the preinjured couple, even though one of the partners may now have become a caretaker. *Sexual Options for Paraplegics and Quadriplegics,* by Mooney, Cole, and Chilgren, gives explicit suggestions for managing catheters and urine bags, as well as

explicit examples of different positions to use for sexual intercourse. This book gives much more specific details about techniques for having sexual activity with disabilities than we can here.
It is also helpful to read, even if you are not disabled but need to
alter your sexual activity as the result of illness. Alternatives are
applicable to any situation.

It is gratifying for most couples to find that once they are able
to talk about these things, they can find all sorts of ways to help
themselves enjoy each other. They can use sexual films, devices,
publications; they are limited only by their personal preferences
and imaginations. There will be a mourning of losses and a sadness
about the sexual activities that are lost. However, there can still
be a sharing of sexual excitement, and the expression of caring
and love for each other. The technical aspects of how to carry out
the sexual activities is the easy part. First each person has to want
to have sex together. Ultimately, it is the emotional quality of
lovemaking that gives each person satisfaction, not the orgasm or
intercourse. If there were problems in the emotional relationship
before the illness or injury, it will only make things that much
more difficult, and outside counseling should be sought.

It is important, as well, to keep religious beliefs in mind. These
could play a role in what a couple feels is acceptable and proper
in sexual activity. Talking with a minister or pastoral counselor
can be helpful to obtain permission to experiment sexually and
relieve guilt.

◆ Kim finally decided to talk to Mike about their sex life. Instead
of Mike's sympathizing with her, he refused to talk about the
problem, and for several days seemed irritated and demanding.
Kim was devastated and resolved not to bring the subject up again.
Besides, her having to attend to his physical needs—like changing
his urine bag, bathing him, and managing his bowel care—made
her feel more like a nurse than a mate.

For spinal-cord injured persons or any other neurologic illness
in which there is loss of the functions of elimination (e.g., some
cases of multiple sclerosis), it is particularly important for the
person to manage his own bowel and bladder needs, if possible,

in order to feel a sense of control over something he/she always had control over. This also helps build confidence that, in the community and in personal relationships, the injured person can handle accidents and his personal needs. If at all possible, wives or husbands should not be expected to do bowel and bladder care. It is very important for the injured or disabled person to retain his privacy and sense of self-esteem. If the spouse does this work, he/she touches a part of the body that also arouses sexual feelings and can be part of sexual acts. In addition, the act of caring for the basic bowel and bladder needs is much like that of a parent caring for an infant; the fact that one of the partners needs this type of help may be perceived as shameful or disgusting, or both. The injured person should do as much as he/she can for himself, with help from aides or nurses. His/her relationship with a partner needs to remain as similar to the preinjury relationship as possible in terms of personal care. Even if the able-bodied spouse does not mind doing this type of care (and many don't), the injured or ill person may feel guilty and feel like a burden. However, if there is no other choice, then being aware of the difficulty of the dual roles of lover and caretaker can be helpful. Talking about the difficulties and feelings each has can make it possible to overcome concerns, and permit this task to be like any other in the ongoing care of the ill or injured person.

When one person becomes irritated and demanding—as Mike does in this vignette, though it does not matter who it is—the other might be alerted that something is wrong and is not being talked about. This needs to be recognized by both parties so that one of the pair does not react by feeling rejected and devastated. If a spouse suspects that their partner is not communicating what they really are feeling or thinking, then it is helpful to initiate a discussion. The "ten-minute" exercise described above should be used whenever it appears that communication has stopped. Each spouse needs to be alerted to those times that they think the other is not talking when they should be. Then they can approach the silent partner and say, "It is time for us to sit down and listen to each other for ten minutes. Let's do it now." A major destroyer of relationships is the use of the silent treatment. This behavior has the effect of pushing a spouse further away and closing all doors to communication. The angry partner is isolated, and the hurt partner is not able to feel sympathetic, because they are so angry and insulted. Nothing feels more frustrating or humiliating, besides physical abuse, to the person being closed out. Rather than get into the vicious cycle of the silent treatment, mutually agree that you will not do that to each other. If you can't talk about things right away, agree to say so to each other. For example, a partner can say, "I will talk with you later. Right now I can't talk about it because I am too angry. Leave me alone for an hour."

◆ After several months, Kim and Mike were finally able to talk about their mutual sexual needs. They had even tried to make love, holding each other and touching. Kim was often excited by the thought of intimacy with her husband, but by the time he was ready—bladder emptied, maneuvered into bed, etc.—she usually found her passion dissipated. She also hated having to look at his lifeless legs; it always reminded her of how athletic he used to be. She hated to see his wheelchair and often felt fearful without apparent cause.

A spouse may not realize that he or she is reacting to the lack of spontaneity and to the mechanical nature of preparing for sex. In addition, if only one of the pair is feeling romantic, the passionate feelings can quickly become embarrassing and pass. If Kim is feeling her passion dissipate, Mike will realize it. Kim may be fearful that she will hurt Mike. It is not uncommon to fear causing more losses to the injured person. It might be helpful to talk with professionals who deal with persons with similar illnesses or injuries to understand better what can and cannot be done physically. There are national and local associations dealing with almost all the major types of illness and neurologic injuries. These organizations usually have a patient services department to answer questions, provide support groups, and visitors to the home-bound. They will have almost certainly faced all the major problems a newly diagnosed or injured person encounters. Books that can also be helpful are *Sexuality and Chronic Illness*, Leslie R. Schover and Soren Buus Jensen; *Sexual Options for Paraplegics and Quadriplegics*, Mooney, Cole, and Chilgren, 1975; *Toward*

Intimacy (Task Force on Concerns of Physically Disabled Women,
1980, and *Arthritis: Living and Loving,* Arthritis Foundation, 1982,
in *Sexuality and Chronic Illness,* 1988. (See Appendix 2.)

Kim's feelings about the wheelchair are also not uncommon,
and reflect her feelings toward the changes the injury has made in
their lives. It was much easier for her to allow herself to hate the
wheelchair than to be angry at her husband and to feel the pain
over his dissipated body. Yet the feelings are there and most likely
have arisen at this time because they now have resumed sexual
activity. Feelings of anger and loss are almost universal in situations like this. Natural as they are, they also almost always lose
their potency to harm the relationship when they are brought out
into the open and discussed. Kim may only now be able to feel
them. Mourning the losses is an essential part of what she and
Mike need to do before they can find that their new ways of
expressing their sexual feelings are satisfying and exciting. As they
continue to experiment, they will regain their previous intimacy
and closeness.

Lisa

◆ Lisa was a junior in college when she first developed inflammatory bowel disease. She had planned to become an elementary
teacher and had hoped to marry and raise a family. At first her
illness responded to drugs and her fiancé, Roy, was very supportive. However, when the illness flared and Lisa spent many weeks
in the hospital, Roy became discouraged. She lost weight and
became haggard-looking. Roy began to visit less and less often.
Finally, the doctors told her she had to have most of her colon
removed and would have a permanent colostomy with an opening
on her abdomen. This was the last straw for Roy, who announced
he could no longer cope with her illness and broke their engagement. After the surgery, Lisa felt physically better, regained weight,
and was able to finish college. However, she had not had any dates
and took little pride in her appearance. She avoided lengthy conversations and closeness, especially with men.

An abnormality relating to the bowels can make the sufferer feel smelly, unclean, and disgusting. As we have mentioned before, each of us has a sexual self-image. We have feelings about our bodies and about how we look to someone else when we are naked. Lisa is having difficulty anticipating that she can be sexually desirable. Roy's leaving the relationship at a time when her self-image is being torn apart does not help her self-esteem, nor does it help her to feel less vulnerable. Some people, like Roy, cannot experience closeness when illness or physical disfigurement is present because it frightens them and reminds them of their own vulnerability and mortality. This kind of rejection can affect the confidence of the ill person for years to come, leaving them feeling that no one will want to be close to them. Ostomy support groups run by self-help organizations or independent ostomy groups can be invaluable to a man or woman in this very common situation. These groups allow people who have the same problem to share and empathize, as well as educate and advise. Lisa could express her feelings of rejection and repulsion and find a sympathetic audience who could also offer advice.

◆ Lisa was able to tell her doctor about some of her concerns, and he referred her to a club composed of colostomy patients. This helped her resolve some of her problems, but she still had difficulty feeling good about herself and could not imagine that a man could ever make love to her the way she was. One day she saw an ad in the personals column of the newspaper. She answered an ad and arranged to meet the man at a local coffee shop. After a short visit, they went to a hotel and had sex. She never saw him again, nor did she want to. Despite her repulsion at this type of intimacy and the type of partners she might encounter, Lisa found herself scanning the newspaper personals column every day for appealing ads. She answered several ads and repeated her one-night-stand experiences several times in the next several months.

Lisa is not ready to take a risk with an eligible partner. She needs to feel that she can still engage in sexual acts and seems to be testing herself. Going to bed with a person she will never see again protects her from rejection and from having to communicate about her physical condition. She is still having some problems with her self-image and still feels vulnerable. There is no danger of feeling hurt or rejected in a series of one-night stands. This can help resolve her fears that no one could make love to someone with such a disfigurement. While this may be necessary in her life right now, this sort of activity, however, won't lead to a lasting, meaningful relationship, which can come only once such feelings are resolved.

◆ After a number of months, Lisa's former easy-going personality began to show, and she began to develop relationships in spite of herself. When she divulged her "secret," she was amazed at how little difference it seemed to make to most people.

Most people, even those with severe injuries or illnesses, are able to regain their previous self-esteem and form relationships with others again. When two people can talk freely together and share feelings about each other, they express closeness and intimacy. They trust each other with knowledge of their imperfections. No one has a perfect body. How one thinks their imperfections are perceived by others and how they are really perceived may be completely different. Lisa might have found her imperfection terrible to contemplate, but a person who liked her enough to date her could find the colostomy simply an annoyance. Relationships have more to do with feeling respected and feeling respect for someone you also feel connected to, sharing experiences, and having companionship, than with our idealized but unrealistic ideas of perfect bodies and beauty. A partner of Lisa's who can help her change her ostomy appliance, demonstrates without a doubt that he finds her sexually attractive. When each person in the relationship can respond so that their partner feels like a sexual being, then there is intimacy. Frequent experiences with men which strengthen her perception that she is sexually attractive will teach Lisa, as it does us all, that she can be loved and have satisfying relationships and sexual encounters.

◆ When erections are sporadic or nonexistent, and when orgasm has been impaired, many people feel sex must be over. That is *not* true.

◆ There is no right way or one way that guarantees sexual satisfaction. Any way that is enjoyable is the right way.

◆ Everytime intimacy is shared, it doesn't have to lead to intercourse. A focus on enjoying each other and enjoying lovemaking can be as satisfying.

◆ Check with your physician to be sure that none of the medications being taken are affecting sexual functioning.

◆ The use of penile implants, dildos, penis stiffeners, etc., are possible, if desired, to enable sexual intercourse.

◆ To help develop problem-solving ability, sit down together for ten minutes. Each person takes a turn speaking for five minutes without being interrupted, while using "I" statements to describe his/her feelings and thoughts about sexuality ("I feel that . . ."). No responses are necessary. It is only necessary to try to understand what the problems are that may be getting in the way of intimacy. After each person has had a turn speaking, list what each thinks the problems are, and look for solutions together.

◆ If the well partner initiates affection, touching, and hugging, it tells the ill or disabled partner that he/she is still sexually attractive.

◆ A major destroyer of affection is the use of the silent treatment.

◆ It is common to fear that the resumption of sexual activity may cause further harm to the ill or disabled person. This is not usually true but needs to be discussed with a physician so that all questions can be answered and fears removed for both partners.

◆ Mourning the losses by talking about feelings is an essential part of what needs to be done so that new ways of expressing sexual feelings can be explored. Sometimes professional counseling can be very helpful in this process.

CHAPTER 13

Understanding Fears of Death

All of us know that we will someday die, but most of us spend little time thinking about it. Nothing brings home one's own mortality like the death of a close relative or friend, or the onset of a potentially fatal illness. Fears of death are extremely common when these events occur, but because of our cultural difficulties in dealing with death, these fears are often disguised and not expressed in ways that are immediately recognizable.

In this chapter, three very common manifestations of the fear of death are explored. Renee, who has a slowly progressive terminal illness, has a recurring nightmare of someone nearly killing her. In the vignette of Sonja and Ty, the fear of dying is expressed as a phobia of being alone, and the affected person requires that someone be with her at all times. This particular expression of the fear of death is particularly common in older persons, and in younger or older persons with terminal illness. It is almost as if by having someone else always present, death cannot enter the premises. In our third example, Gerta is prepared for death, but her son is not, as he is the one who is having problems dealing with it.

There is no easy way to deal with such fears, but understanding that the experiences one is having really represent such fears can sometimes make them easier to live with.

Renee

◆ Renee was a career woman. Early in her working life she had in effect chosen her accounting career over her marriage and had divorced while still in her twenties. Now in her late forties, she had achieved a good deal of success, but it had been at a price. She had devoted many hours each day to her job and had formed few close friends; she had dealt with the stresses of the job by chain smoking. A few months ago she had noticed shortness of breath climbing stairs, and it had been gradually getting worse. Her doctor told her that she had emphysema and that stopping smoking would slow the progression of the disease, but that she would continue to get worse. She listened to him but decided she would be an old woman before the emphysema slowed her down. Initially she tried to stop smoking but found it very difficult and finally gave up. Recently she had been having another problem which was very distressing and occupied her mind even at work. She had had recurrent dreams of someone choking her and letting her go just before she passed out. In the last few nights, she was so frightened of having the dream again, that she put off going to bed until very late and then became very anxious and had difficulty breathing. This would cause her to panic, which made her more short of breath. It was sometimes fifteen or twenty minutes before she could get ahold of herself; she was becoming a nervous wreck.

During serious illness or other crises, the human mind and body work together to control or make manageable, strong debilitating feelings. The fears one has can be so overwhelming that the mind will not allow the feelings to be felt and experienced. It is an internal means of protecting the organism. At these times the feelings are suppressed and can reappear as otherwise unexplainable symptoms or frightening dreams.

Renee's dream is an example of how fears can be expressed in dreams. Her dream appears as an expression of her fear of dying, which at present she cannot express any other way. It may be that her fear of choking is related to her knowledge about emphysema—nothing is quite so terrifying as feeling you cannot get your breath. Just thinking about the idea of not being able to breathe

BUILDING A NEW DREAM

can bring on anxiety and panic. The fact is that breathing for Renee is now difficult, and in the future will become more difficult for her.

Before she will be able to understand the dreams, it will be necessary for her to recognize that they represent her fear of death. This will require a good deal of insight; it may be necessary for a professional counselor to help her correctly interpret her dreams and her reactions to them. Sometimes though, we are able to understand our dreams without outside help and realize what we are worrying about. At these times, it can be helpful to seek out friends or family members to talk with about it.

Her difficulty giving up cigarettes in the face of so serious an illness suggests an underlying conflict. Recognizing the meaning of her nightmares and the fears they embody would help Renee confront the fact that she needs to make some changes in her life-style. Then she can begin learning how to cope with these changes and her illness. These changes could increase her functioning and possibly slow down the progression of her illness.

It is time for Renee to look at her goals for the future. She has devoted much of her life to work, which has been a satisfying and rewarding outlet for her. But she may not be able to continue her work much longer in a fulfilling way, and she may want to look at how to increase satisfaction in other areas. It is not too late to do this. Thus her fears are fortuitously providing her with an opportunity both to talk about her dreams and feelings of panic with a professional, to begin changing her perception of herself and her life-style, and to plan for the future. Once these things are in the open and obvious to her, Renee will be able to see the connection between her feelings, her illness, and the way she has lived her life. This will help to alleviate the anxiety and panic, and allow her to plan ways to stop smoking, slow down at work, and begin to have some recreation and other people in her life. Because she is scared, Renee has motivation to think about why she is still smoking and why she has turned to work rather than people so much. If she cannot begin to change some of these behaviors by herself, then with help she can.

Panic and anxiety often accompany serious illnesses, especially illnesses such as emphysema in which breathing is affected.

Relaxation-training techniques reduce panic and lower levels of anxiety. Renee can learn these techniques from a professional trained in behavioral techniques (see Chapter 5: Finding and Using Community Resources, on locating the correct professional help) and use them throughout the day prior to feeling panic and anxiety, as well as to control anxiety attacks when they occur. These techniques can be learned quickly, in about ten sessions. Professionals use muscle tension and relaxation, deep breathing, or imagery to teach people how to relax and control anxiety. It is not possible to be both anxious and relaxed at the same time. So for controlling anxiety, relaxation training can be very effective. (See also Chapter 9: Managing Personality Changes.)

After a diagnosis of a serious illness, fears of death are common. Most times our characteristic ways of handling fears help us cope. Often the fear that one feels after hearing a diagnosis of life-threatening illness helps motivate helpful and permanent life-style changes. Denial, though, can occur. (That is, acting as if one did not have a life-threatening illness that needs attention.) Denial is frequently a useful way to cope, as long as the changes necessary to help increase longevity and constructive planning for the future occur. If denial is excessive and hampers the person or his family from even slowly coming to terms with the illness and making the necessary life-style changes to minimize the effects of the problem, friends or family might try to help the person see a professional for help in adapting and coping. Sometimes all well-meaning efforts to get the ill or disabled to talk about their fears or change unhealthy behaviors fail. The denial becomes excessive, and the dysfunctional behaviors don't change. There is very little that anyone can do when that happens. The ill or disabled have to take some responsibility for their lives. Sometimes only after further losses or another acute episode, does the ill or disabled person admit that he has to change his life-style. This is hard on the family, but sometimes it is the only way.

Sonja and Ty

◆ Sonja's seizures started after a minor car accident in which she had hit her head against the window and suffered a concussion.

They were quite well controlled with medication, but occasionally she had one which consisted of her losing consciousness, falling to the floor, and having jerking movements of her arms and legs for about a minute. Then she would have a period of several minutes before she woke up. The seizures only happened once every few months, but since they had started Sonja had undergone a marked change which neither she nor her husband Ty liked very much. Before the accident, Sonja had handled all the affairs of the household including shopping, maintenance, finances, day-to-day crises. Now she was terrified of being alone—ever. It made no sense either to her or Ty. She always had a sense of when a seizure was about to occur and could protect herself from harm by lying down. Yet she was so frightened of being alone that she was afraid to go to sleep at night. Her fear was frightening to Ty, too, and he did not like leaving her when she felt like that. In order to go to work, Ty had had to hire an attendant to stay with her all day; he had not had a night out with the boys since the accident and was beginning to feel like a caged animal. Besides that, having to pay for an attendant was straining their finances.

The reaction Sonja is having is very common in victims of serious illness or illness with frightening and unpredictable symptoms. Such intense fears of being alone can be related to a number of concerns: a fear of harm, a sense of helplessness over one's fate, a fear of dying alone, or a fear of becoming more disabled and nonfunctioning.

A closely related fear is that if the person participates in any activity, a worsening of the condition or a repeat of unpleasant symptoms may result. This causes noncompliance and inactivity. For example, a patient may be hesitant to participate in a rehabilitation program for fear of precipitating either another stroke, a seizure, a worse spinal injury, or exacerbating a multiple sclerosis episode, etc., that will then result in further and worse disability. If these fears are not recognized and articulated, then they might be expressed through severe anxiety and dependency. Whenever you act in a way that seems irrational or counterproductive, stop and ask yourself, "Why did I do that?" You can almost always find a previously unrecognized reason to account for your actions; this is how you gain insight into your behavior.

Sonja, in this example, may fear dying or harming herself further if she were to fall and hit her head. Some of her fears might also be related to early family experiences with relatives or close family members who made fun of or ridiculed people who suffered seizures from epilepsy.

Such fears can have a major impact on the life of a spouse. When a spouse sees the ill person afraid of being alone, he/she feels the person's vulnerability and this makes them feel compelled to stay. Indeed, they may have their own fears about their loved one dying or being alone if something happened. This has the net effect of preventing them from participating in those activities that they enjoy and find relaxing, or meeting their personal responsibilities.

Hiring an attendant gives Ty some time off, but it is not a solution to the underlying problem in this case. If Ty shares Sonja's fear that something will happen to her, this fear will prevent practical solutions for help or respite. Typically, the spouses do not discuss these things. The well spouse becomes exhausted and isolated but unable not to be with his wife. Yet, ironically, the time spent together is almost totally centered on the illness, not on their relationship or each other.

A common misconception is that talking about these things will be embarrassing or hurtful to the ill person. Talking is the *only* way to start toward a solution. Whatever the specific fears are for Sonja (or anyone who feels as she does about being alone), she would be greatly helped if she could talk about her fears. Sometimes talking about what you fear, even if it seems embarrassing or silly, can be reassuring. In fact, often the person who is affected does not really realize that he has a paralzying fear; he just knows that he cannot bear the thought of being alone. Talking may enable him to give form to this feeling and recognize it as a fear. Saying what seems so unspeakable often is very relieving in and of itself. For example, the husband in this example might initiate a conversation by saying, "What is it, Sonja, that you are feeling when I get ready to leave?" She might answer, "I really do not know. I never thought about putting it into words. It is almost too painful to put into words. It is almost as if someone were clutching my heart and squeezing the life out of me. It's terrifying." Sonja has now come closer to crystallizing her thoughts and recognizing her feelings as an irrational fear. Now she may be able to start dealing with the feelings. Unfortunately, it is not always possible for a spouse to initiate conversations like this. If this approach is unsuccessful, Sonja may need a brief period of professional counseling to confront her fears. Another alternative is that of self-help groups that deal with unreasonable fears or with seizure disorders. These can be contacted through local mental-health societies, local hospitals, and local branches of associations that are set up to deal with specific illnesses.

Many misconceptions can be corrected as a result of subsequent conversations or subsequent information seeking, which follow the difficult initial conversations about fears and worries; and then plans can be made that meet both person's needs. The worst problem that occurs in families is when things do not get talked about. Everyone unintentionally and helplessly colludes in what seems like a conspiracy of silence. To help Sonja and Ty open up, family members can approach them and ask if they are worried or if they would like to talk. Ty has made some decisions without discussing them with his wife. Unilateral decisions based on what the well person making the decision thinks is good for the other person, are unfair to the ill person. Here again, great progress could be obtained if other family members could speak to the couple or if they could speak to each other.

Gerta

◆ Gerta was old and she had cancer of her colon. She had lived a long life without misgivings and felt ready to die. In a strange way she felt lucky that as her death approached, she still had a clear mind and could make her own decisions. When the cancer began to ravage her body and she began to lose weight, her appetite also failed. She was grateful that the cancer was not causing pain, but she knew that eventually it would and that would make each remaining day of her life agony. She would rather die now before the disease robbed her of her dignity, and so she decided to stop eating. Her son, Manny, watched this course of events with great distress. He could not bear the sight of her wasting away and took her from doctor to doctor in vain attempts to find some way to get her to start eating again.

Manny's reasons for wanting to keep his mother alive are several. He will of course miss her and feel great grief at the loss, but he also does not want to have to confront the reality and finality of death as he will when she dies. Manny in part is attempting to keep Gerta alive because of his own fears about death and mortality. When someone we love chooses death over life, it may feel as if they do not care about those of us left behind. It is as if they are saying that we are not important enough to them for them to go on living. This hurts and sometimes makes us angry, even though it may have nothing to do with the reasons they made the decision to die.

To deal with his own fears of death, a child or other surviving person may put great effort into vain attempts at saving the dying person's life. It is much more difficult to respect the dying person's decision and mourn with them. This usually results in frustration and distress for everyone, and it is expensive as well! The task for family members is to come to terms with the fact that someone they love is dying. In this vignette, Manny needs to find a way that is comfortable for him to say goodbye to his mother. Talking with Gerta about her life, her decision, or anything else which would allow them to comfort each other, would be a special gift and what Manny should do.

One of the advantages of respecting the wishes of the dying person is that it allows people to share some very important feelings. There may be people Gerta would like to see. There may be some unfinished business and unfinished relationships that she might want to finish. If Manny is able to, he can help Gerta finish old business. The sense of having things in order, and of saying goodbye, brings peace. Manny's obvious love for his mother can be expressed verbally and positively rather than by a fruitless search for a nonexistent reprieve from the illness. There are frequently many things not said to people we love that later we wish we had said. There are so many unnecessary, unspoken rules

202   BUILDING A NEW DREAM

against sharing feelings, pain, or happiness. If Manny wants to and can put aside his fears, he has an opportunity to try things in a new way here. He can talk to his mother about her life and his. He can find out all the things he wanted to know about her past and his heritage. He can help her die with dignity and with love. No, this usually cannot be done without tears. You both feel sad about the impending end of your relationship, but you also feel good about being able to end it the best possible way. It is OK to cry; when people are sad, they cry.

However, not every family wants to or can express these kinds of feelings. If the family members are unable to talk about their feelings, it is still helpful to know that the unspoken, underlying emotions often represent a fear of one's own death and the fear and sadness over the loss of a beloved family member. For many people, fighting to keep a loved one alive allows them to feel that they did everything possible to save the person and this can allow them to feel at peace after the person dies.

◆ Most chronically ill persons are subconsciously afraid they will die soon, but these feelings are so painful they are often disguised as recurrent nightmares or the need to have someone else always with them.

◆ Bringing the fears and feelings out into the open is the only way to confront and remove such unpleasant experiences and needs. However, since these emotions are so powerful, this may be difficult to do, and professional counseling may be necesssary.

◆ Sometimes an adult child's fear of his parent's death is so strong that it prevents him from visiting the parent or talking with him/her about death. If the child can recognize and come to terms with his emotions, he will be able to share important feelings and say goodbye.

THREE

Social Consequences
of Illness

CHAPTER 14

Handling Changes at Work

One of the first crises an unexpected illness can precipitate is difficulties at the workplace. Employers are often skittish about sick employees and concerned about the impact on their costs, like health insurance, as well as the productivity of the employee. Even though many such fears are unfounded, if one adds to them the afflicted person's own doubts about his ability to perform, the result can be overwhelming stress that spills over into the person's and the family's private lives. The vignettes in this chapter illustrate some common issues regarding one's work, which can arise when a chronic illness occurs.

Gerald, who has had a heart attack, and Marie, his wife, illustrate a couple in the midst of productive life with two children to support and many upcoming expenses, including university costs. This couple, besides suffering the emotional and physical impact of serious disease at a relatively young age, must face financial hardship because of a loss of earning power.

Maggie is a single woman nearing retirement, whose whole life has been devoted to her work. She develops a sudden severe disability when a car accident results in paralysis. As if her problems are not enough, she then develops delayed progressive nerve loss secondary to her injury. Loss of work for her, in effect, takes away a major part of her life and is devastating.

Everett faces a quite different problem. He develops occupational asthma, a medical condition related to his work environment that makes it impossible for him to continue in that type of job. The potential consequences financially, especially for someone skilled in a particular area, can be profound. Fortunately, in work-related illness, help in financial compensation and retraining is often available and will be discussed.

Finally, in Liann's case she has an illness, diabetes mellitus, which presently has no impact on her work. However, the potential complications of the illness, now twenty years from its onset, might require her to have time-consuming treatments that will affect her ability to continue her job. How can one work around time commitments like this, or is it necessary to give up employment in such a situation?

You may find yourself in a situation similar to one of these. In the discussion we will offer approaches to coping with stressful circumstances arising out of one's workplace, and ways to handle changes that might be necessary in one's work.

Gerald and Marie

◆ Gerald and Marie worked very hard to provide a good life for themselves and sons Dino, 17, and Don, 15. In fact Gerald had at times held down two construction jobs simultaneously and was popularly referred to by friends as a workaholic. He did everything intensely, including eating, and was about forty pounds overweight. Thus it was more of a surprise to Gerald than his coworkers when one morning he developed chest pains at work. The heart attack that followed kept him off the job for a month, but he was chomping at the bit to get back to work—and he wasn't very easy to live with at home either. Finally, with a great deal of badgering, his doctor agreed to let him return to the job. When Gerald returned to his job, which involved moving heavy blocks for building house foundations, he found things a bit different. He fatigued easily and, at times, even though he was taking medication, would feel a heaviness in his chest that frightened him. Before the heart attack he was one of the best in the trade and this was important to him; but now it was clear—to his great disappointment and shame—that he was having difficulty keeping up with others. He became concerned that he might get fired.

The first time the emotional impact really hits home may be when it becomes necessary to really make the changes in all aspects of one's life, including one's work, which a serious life-threatening illness requires. The workplace must be viewed from several perspectives. It provides a social world as well as a sense of identity. Providing for one's family brings a sense of self-worth and a sense of productivity. It is important to feel that one is making a contribution to society. Work-related changes bring their own set of fears about financial losses, loss of respect, and loss of a sense of self-worth. Gerald's initial reaction of fear and shame is common. It is also common for the person to suppress these feelings and not discuss them with his wife or coworkers. This often leads to the person's denying that any changes at all at work have to be made. The overall result is to delay a satisfactory adjustment to returning to work if limitations now exist. Unfortunately, before the person will allow himself to face the new restrictions, in an effort to prove himself—or to reaffirm to himself that he still is capable of doing the job—he may place himself in a position, by trying to go back to work, where it is even more apparent that he cannot do the job anymore. This leads to more stress before he can come to terms with his new status and cope satisfactorily. It is hard to talk a person out of this who has a lot of pride and wants to prove he can still do the job. But every effort should be made to encourage the person to speak with his/her boss about new responsibilities early in recovery. A spouse or family member can be very helpful in this. For example, a brother, uncle, cousin, etc., right before Gerald returns to work, can sit down with him and say, "Listen, Gerald, I know you think you are going to go right back to work as if nothing has happened. But think about it first. OK? Talk to your boss about other work you can do. You don't have to prove anything to us. We know you. Don't overdo it. We don't want to lose you." Also spouses or close relatives can talk to bosses for the ill or disabled person, asking a boss to talk to the ill person upon his return. Sometimes the ill or disabled person is grateful for this kind of assistance, and it makes it easier to talk to their boss.

The first step toward a good and positive adjustment—and one which can eliminate unnecessary further emotional pain—is the early recognition of certain work limitations. Sometimes these are not known in advance, and the best approach is to start back at a less strenuous job and gradually work up to whatever capacity is manageable. This approach can greatly reduce the panic, shame, and embarrassment one might feel if he starts back at too difficult a job and fails at it. It is also an approach which is understood and accepted both by coworkers and employers.

In a new, sudden-onset illness you should, of course, discuss in detail with the physician caring for you when to return to work and in what capacity. Bear in mind, however, that a physician will often give you general guidelines, but you will be the only one who can judge just what your capabilities and limitations will be, and you must be honest with yourself about this. Only you know if you are becoming overly fatigued or are experiencing chest pains, etc.

Another situation often faced in chronic illness is that of gradually decreasing capability (rather than a sudden loss of capability). Again, the first and most important step is to discuss with the doctor what one's capabilities ought to be and then apply this to one's own work situation.

Sometimes it may be necessary to give up a job because of the limitations resulting from illness or disability. This at times depends on the nature of the work and the willingness of both the ill person and the employer to discuss possible alternatives to the current job responsibilities. Thus, before making a decision to relinquish a position, the ill person needs to have a frank discussion with the boss. This can lead to many alternatives. Companies often are willing to decrease hours or days or make work roles less physically demanding. Options for bosses are multiple. For example, a valued employee with specific knowledge and experience might well become a resource person for training others or for supervising. This could allow a shift from physically demanding jobs to more sedentary ones. For this sort of adjustment to be satisfactory, it is necessary to find out and recognize early an accurate estimation of the degree of limitation. As already mentioned, the first step is a forthright discussion with the doctor and then with the employer so that everyone—including you—has a realistic impression of what one can or cannot do.

Keeping in mind that work roles can be adapted or altered for ill or disabled employees reduces the emotionally crippling effects of panic and fear of failure that may make one's limitations seem greater than they really are! An honest appraisal of one's capabilities is of critical importance to the well-being of the whole family. Knowing that despite job changes one can still be a contributor to the family helps to reduce fears of financial disaster and loss of love.

When adjustments are difficult or major changes in jobs are necessary, family members or even the ill person might entertain and encourage the idea of retirement. Unless the person is already near retirement age or has severe disability, however, this is usually not the best option. The ability to contribute financially to the family and gain some satisfaction from his work allows a person an irreplaceable sense of well-being and self-worth. Nothing is more effective then to maintain important roles, such as work roles, in the event of illness. This helps to avoid or lessen depression and anxiety over the losses due to the illness. Furthermore, giving up a job often has wide-ranging effects beyond the immediate emotional and financial. A whole family may suffer from loss of future pension, life and health insurance, profit-sharing plans, or a whole range of other benefits enjoyed by most employees. For all these reasons, then, premature retirement, unless forced by the degree of physical limitation or the employer, should not be encouraged.

◆ At the urging of his wife, who was greatly concerned about Gerald's deepening distress over his inadequacies at work and his eroding self-esteem, Gerald finally visited his doctor for a careful assessment of his capabilities. The heavy work, the doctor confirmed, was now too physically demanding with Gerald's damaged heart; however, Gerald would be able to continue in the construction industry in a lighter job. The doctor would supply whatever documentation was necessary, both requesting a less strenuous job and affirming that Gerald could safely work in such a less demanding position.

We feel that a few more thoughts might be helpful for those who must decrease their workloads because it is so difficult for many of us to accept this, especially when we have worked very hard to get to our present positions and are very proud of our achievements. Many men and women—though often the cultural pressures on men are greater—can make the adjustments necessary, but embarrassment and pride prevent them from speaking to their bosses and seeking less demanding work. It can be a matter of bruised self-esteem and the fear of appearing that one is not on a par with one's peers. In explaining a change in jobs, many men and women (sometimes to their own surprise) find themselves telling their peers they have either been promoted or have lost interest in their old job, rather than have to admit that they need to work at a less demanding job because of illness.

It might help to understand that this behavior is not so much a reflection of the ill person's character as a reflection of the society in which he lives. In North American society, weakness is bad. Competition is fierce and there is a constant battle to never appear "down one" with peers. Illness, which represents weakness, can be perceived as an evil force on one's family and as such makes the ill person a loser. Discussing such common fears with one's family and one's physician is in effect admitting to them and— yes, it is true—that helps relieve the anxiety.

It is not really necessary to tell your workmates all the details of your life. If it helps to find other reasons for important work-related decisions, then so be it. But it is important for you to recognize why you are giving the reasons that you are for your job change. If you do not, you may become so worried about people finding out the real reason that the stress affects your already compromised health. The other danger to watch out for is the sense of being overly stigmatized or uncompetitive, so that withdrawal and apathy develop. If this happens, you should seek some help in adapting and coping from a physician or other counselor. (See Chapter 7: Coping with Depression.)

◆ With the help of his doctor and frank discussions with his employer, Gerald, who had fifteen years of experience with the company, was given an administrative position in the company. Unfortunately, he now had a straight salary and no overtime and this resulted in a big drop in his (and his family's) income. So now he had new worries. Though he had finished paying off the house last year, he was now facing college tuition for his two boys and knew he could not cover that expense with his new earnings.

Being able to continue to contribute financially to the family certainly helps avoid financial crisis and lessens some of the emotional turmoil. It would be unrealistic, though, to believe that keeping a job, albeit modified, will prevent all stress. Job modifications may mean lower salaries; a reduction in the number of hours or days worked means less take-home pay at the same salary. And these financial changes, if no other income is available, will likely mean a changed life-style for the whole family.

Family members may feel resentful that their standard of living has declined and subconsciously and irrationally blame the ill person; the person himself will certainly feel this tension and in turn experience guilt and fears about the security of his family. Even with the absence of any family resentment, he may feel like a failure to the family and worry about the family's security, which spouses and children may have difficulty understanding.

Often an ill person will not volunteer such feelings because of the pride attached to a work role and the subsequent difficulty in accepting necessary changes. Family members may need to ask about such feelings as the ill person is often reluctant to bring them up. It is important for family members to acknowledge these feelings and to recognize that they are common human responses and not to be ashamed of them. One way to do this is for family members to sit down together and talk openly about the differences in life-style that will now be necessary, and discuss their reactions about these changes. If they find the modifications in life-style difficult to accept, together they can decide on a plan to lessen the impact of their financial losses. Children or other family members may well come up with suggestions that the parents have not thought of! An example in this particular case might be that the child will choose a less expensive college than he had planned for.

Most couples can talk about their disappointments and make the necessary life-style adjustments. But if this does not happen and resentment builds so that there is a lot of family conflict, it may become necessary to get some professional help to talk openly about these feelings.

Everyone's financial situation is different, and at a time of financial crisis, each family needs to make a point of taking time to take a careful look at its sources of income. Planning for the future is critical. If no one in the family is skilled at financial matters, professional financial help may be worth the cost because of the need for careful planning.

It is important to investigate all possible resources. If one owns a home, a cooperative apartment, or a condominium apartment, these assets may be used as equity. It might be possible to rent space in one's home or to create space in one's home to rent. Educational loans for the children may be necessary to help them complete their educations. Life or other insurance policies should be checked to see if there is a provision for disability income; loan agreements should be reviewed to see if there is insurance that pays them off in the event of serious disability of the loanee. Private partial disability policies, workmen's compensation, and government Social Security or insurance plans may provide some funds. Unions sometimes have funds to help disabled members who have financial losses due to changes in work responsibilities, as do other types of organizations. Assets must be catalogued: insurance plans, savings accounts, stocks and bonds, real estate, and personal property such as automobiles.

Someone else in the household may have to get a job. This may be the spouse or the older children. Teenagers can often find part-time work. This could help as long as it is very necessary and they really want to do it. However, it is important to strike a balance here. Dropping out of school to work full-time to meet financial obligations will almost always be a cause of future regret, and it may be better to accept a somewhat lower standard of living for a few years to ensure a more secure future. Remember that these are major decisions that will influence the life of everyone in the family. Major family schisms can inadvertently occur if discussions are not handled openly and with everyone's participation. Here are some suggestions to help families get through this period.

The ill person should be included in all discussions where new sources of income are being investigated. It must be recognized by him/her and other family members that if others take jobs, their roles at home will necessarily be reduced. A forum should be arranged (e.g., a regular weekly meeting at a specified time) so that family members can review the new arrangements and decide whether they are working satisfactorily. Or if not, decide how things can be changed.

This is a time that can actually be healing for the whole family and help them to adapt to unfortunate, but as they usually discover, manageable circumstances. Families can join together at these times to help the ill person maintain modifications in his work without unnecessary guilt or sadness, and to help each other deal with their resentments and losses. If spouses and children can be reassuring about the changes in life-style and encouraging about the importance of the ill person maintaining a job, the early shame and panic can be relieved and healthy adaptation can occur. Openly acknowledging each other's contributions can help get everyone through a rough period. Compliment the ill or disabled person for hanging in there and making the necessary changes. The ill or disabled person needs to compliment his family for working with him to find alternative ways to find money and problem solve. Give each other compliments whenever you can.

◆ By utilizing many of the suggestions above, Gerald's family was able to adapt to their new financial status. They all seemed to be settling into the new life-style and were so involved with their own routines, that they did not notice Gerald's increasing withdrawal from family affairs. Finally one evening everyone was forced to recognize that something was amiss because he refused to eat dinner with the family—the one time together he had always insisted on since the children were babies.

The loss of one's work or status through his work is not unlike the loss of a valued relationship with another person or even the loss of a family member or friend. Gerald is experiencing grief at the loss of his work role and that part of him that was expressed through the job. He is mourning just as he might mourn the loss of a life. People often do not recognize that this kind of mourning can occur at losses other than loss of life, and when it does occur, they cannot figure out what is happening to them. It is actually quite a common occurrence.

Why would someone have this type of reaction to the loss of his job? We often do not recognize how important our work is to us until we can no longer do it. For many of us, work is a source of pride through which we can achieve praise and admiration for what we accomplish; it is a source of pride because it allows us to be in control of our lives and allows us to provide for the welfare of our families. Many people find it a source of pride to be able to provide through hard work, opportunities for their children that were not available to them.

Work is a social network. Often friends from work represent our primary social interactions. Friends at work may interact with each other in ways that are entirely different from the ways they interact with family members or any other social contacts. These interactions may be vital, and losing these relationships can be very painful.

People are often unaware that work can be so important a part of one's life. It is often taken for granted as just part of our daily routine. Once we recognize the importance of work, it is easier to see that its loss may cause great grief in the ill person, and the mourning that follows may result in withdrawal and apathy. If the ill person and his family recognize this, they can reassure each other that this process is normal. Finding ways to show the grieving person that he/she is appreciated by the family may ease the process as well. Giving him jobs around home to do, asking his advice, and expressing concern over withdrawal from family affairs are ways to let the ill person know he is important within the family.

Maggie

◆ Maggie was a vice president in the public relations firm where she had worked for many years and was proud of this achievement. In fact, when she was younger she had devoted herself to her work to the extent that she socialized little. She had never developed a network of friends outside of work, nor had she married. How ironic it seemed that on the way to the one party she dutifully attended each year—the company Christmas party—her car was struck broadside by a truck. After several weeks in the hospital, it was clear that she would regain only partial use of her legs; a wheelchair would become a necessity. At age fifty-five, how could she cope with this devastating change in her physical health? She felt she could still do her work, which depended mostly on her hands and mind, but how would she manage the sheer effort of getting from one place to another, let alone in and out of her apartment. She could not even sit at her desk in a wheelchair!

Many illnesses and injuries cause physical limitations that might not in and of themselves impair one's ability to do his job. However, a great deal more is usually involved in the adaptations that victims of arthritis, stroke, spinal-cord injury, multiple sclerosis, Parkinson's Disease, other neurologic diseases, emphysema, and many other illnesses must make to be able to continue their jobs. When physical limitations occur, simply getting to and from work and about the office become major obstacles.

Whether or not Maggie must give up her job does depend on how willing her employer is to make the necessary work-related changes or adaptations. Some employers may want Maggie to retire. Disability insurance, unions, and workmen's compensation need to be checked into to see what financial support is available. Employers' concerns that their workmen's compensation will increase if they retain a disabled employee are not grounded. Workmen's Compensation Second Injury law provides that no increase to the employer for worker's compensation will occur. (See *Na-*

tional Resource Directory, Barry Corbet, editor, National Spinal Cord Injury Association.)

Maggie's boss may be willing to arrange for a desk or buy a desk that would allow her to sit in her wheelchair. Ramps may need to be built to allow access into the building. Bathrooms also need to be wide enough to enter. Maggie may be able to hire an attendant who can help her at home in the evenings. Hand controls would allow her to continue driving. Maggie should go through a rehabilitation program if she is now confined to a wheelchair. She will learn how to be independent in the wheelchair. As the result of her disability, she is entitled to the services of the Division of Vocational Rehabilitation. (See Chapter 5: Finding and Using Community Resources.) Rehabilitation is very important as well for stroke and arthritis victims, and persons suffering from heart disease, emphysema, or bronchitis. In fact for nearly any disease which has physical disability associated with it, there are techniques which can be learned through rehabilitation programs that will greatly help the sufferers get through normal daily routines. Simple things like getting dressed in the morning can seem like mountains to climb for persons with these diseases.

◆ Many changes were made to accommodate Maggie's physical limitations, and initially she was able to carry on her work without undue difficulty. Then, an unfortunate thing happened; she began to have increasing loss of the function of her hands because of a delayed loss of nerve tissue. How could she cope with this new development?

Maggie was unprepared for the progression of her injury. Unpredictable illnesses are very stressful; just as one gets adjusted to his/her limitations, there are a whole new set of obstacles to face. This uncertainty is exhausting. Adjustment is much harder when new deficits occur that were unexpected. If at all possible, unpredictability should be reduced to a minimum by getting as many facts from the doctor as possible about the likely course of the illness right at the beginning. Most people and physicians do not want to be negative. But it is very difficult and really much more frustrating to make plans for the future and then find these plans did not allow for further losses and increased disability. Diseases like multiple sclerosis and Parkinson's Disease, for example, afford no certainty about the progression of the illness; strokes and spinal-cord injuries usually represent unchanging limitations. It may be much harder for patients with multiple sclerosis or Parkinson's Disease to plan for the future as a result.

Moves into new homes or new jobs are decisions that have to take into account the progression of the illness. It is not clear when stairs will become a problem or when there will no longer be two incomes to pay for the expenses. Climate changes from hot to cold or wet to dry might also now have to be taken into account. Snow and ice may pose problems in mobility.

The best way to deal with uncertainty is to plan for it as much as possible. With illnesses like multiple sclerosis or Parkinson's Disease, when it is known that further disability is possible, alternatives made ahead of time can give the family a sense of control. Making two sets of plans in case things change and the illness progresses leads to less disappointment. Another avenue is to prepare for the time when the illness progresses and the disability worsens, by discussing with family members or vocational counselors the kinds of work one might do as the illness progresses. Preparing for retirement and Social Security disability as well as preparing for activities which one will be able to continue to participate in despite further losses can help avoid depression and frustration later.

Sometimes a decision to get early retraining for a more appropriate job if illnesses are likely to progress, or a decision to make an early change of jobs to get experience in another field, will be necessary. It must also be remembered that there are many ways to be productive. A person suffering from retinitis pigmentosa knows he will suffer progressive visual loss. While he may be a commercial artist and successful at it, in ten years he will not be able to continue in his profession though he is still relatively young. Going to see a vocational counselor for career counseling would help him identify possible careers for the future for which eyesight would not be as imperative as it is for the job of a commercial artist. Career counseling and job training are also provided by the Office of Vocational Rehabilitation. (See Chapter 5: Finding and Using Community Resources.)

If retirement becomes necessary, ways can be found to allow the person to continue to be productive. Volunteering can be a very rewarding contribution to society. Doing chores around the house, helping to prepare and plan for family outings, making family decisions, and attending family and community functions are very important and prevent feelings of uselessness and isolation when disabilities become severe. The important thing for families as well as the ill person to remember is that with imagination and the use of assistive devices and equipment, one can find ways to keep productive.

Maggie may be very scared about her future and feel very angry at the sudden and progressive changes. If she takes a chance to talk openly about her fears and her disappointments and explores the resources, services, and programs that are available in the community and which could allow her to continue working and being productive, she could adapt well.

♦ Telephone, word processor, and other adaptations were made in an effort to accommodate Maggie's increasing physical limitations. For two years things went pretty well. However, gradually she began to find it very fatiguing and difficult to carry on her job and felt that her work was not up to par; worse, she felt she was being indulged because of her long years of service. In a sense, she felt trapped and wished she could quit.

We have stressed previously the importance of continuing to work whenever possible, especially when the work is a major part of one's life or the ill person has a provider role in the family. But there are times when it is more important to consider the quality of life one is living. When the mere effort of going to work is tiring and one's quality of work is not up to his/her expectations, the job can become more frustrating than satisfying. At this point, it is easy to become bitter and angry, and retirement, especially for those near retirement age, may be a good option. This is a time to arrange a family meeting to discuss financial needs and make specific plans for retirement. Pension programs, as well as disability insurance plans, either through unions at the job or through Social Security (Social Security Disability Insurance and/or Supplemental Security Income) need to be explored.

Another good option to consider is a move to a warmer climate that would make living in a wheelchair easier, provide money from the sale of a primary residence, and provide more options for recreation. Of course this kind of a move has to take into account the difficulty of being separated from family and friends. Sometimes it is very hard to leave close friends and family behind. There is a sense of security in familiar neighborhoods that develops over the years. Also one develops a network of people one can rely on in emergencies. Leaving this behind frequently results in feelings of depression and requires readaptation to a new place. When one's devotion has been to work and not to interpersonal relationships (as in Maggie's case), moves such as this are easier.

Retirement should not automatically be interpreted as one's loss of usefulness to society. People who feel that they want to continue to be productive can often offer volunteer services on a part-time basis. One often welcome option is to offer to advise, counsel, or assist persons who have recently suffered similar illnesses or injuries. Those who become involved in this type of activity may be pleasantly surprised to find that actual payment for services or the creation of a product is not necessary to make one feel fulfilled.

It is not necessary to feel trapped. It is always possible to sit down and take stock of one's options. Considering alternative lifestyles can increase mood and optimism and lead to more satisfying choices.

Everett

◆ Everett, twenty-eight, had begun to notice something very peculiar over the last few months. Shortly after he arrived at work each morning, he began to cough and feel short of breath. In fact the only time he felt he could breathe comfortably anymore was on weekends and after he'd been on vacation for a few days. He could not understand what was happening. He had been a baker for six years since he had taken over the family business. There was a lot of flour around, but it had never seemed to bother him before. He really felt comfortable with the business now and since it was doing really well, he was thinking of expanding soon. The breathing finally became such a problem that Everett's wife, Joan, made him visit the family doctor. The doctor told Everett he had asthma, and by his history, it was likely due to the flours in the bakery; the only way to prevent the problem would be to get out of the bakery completely. Everett saw his promising, future business disappearing before his eyes; he was despondent.

Everett is a good candidate for the services of the State Division of Vocational Rehabilitation (see Chapter 5: Finding and Using Community Resources). He is a young man and can be helped either to buy a new business or to be retrained for different employment. He will have some immediate losses and emotional turmoil, and possibly some financial difficulty, but he cannot remain in this occupation, and with assistance, he should be able to get back on his feet in a relatively short period of time. Financial help is often available for those with proven occupation-related illness. Most state and provincial governments provide medical and occupational rehabilitation services.

Everett will need to adjust emotionally to the need for a career change. His despondency is reasonable and normal. If he can acknowledge and express his sense of loss and anger over the changes that he must now make to carry on with his life, he can move forward and take advantage of retraining, or selling his business and beginning a new one. It is very hard to accept that the work you loved and put so much energy and hope into developing, could make you sick. It is hard not to be angry and despondent about that. However, the qualities which made Everett successful in the first place, the business acumen, the drive to succeed, and the energy to work hard will always be there. As a result, he can make a success out of another type of business. After a period of sadness, anger, and grieving, planning for a new future direction is the next step. Agencies and services like those described above can be very helpful throughout this process.

Liann

◆ Liann has a disease that afflicts millions of people, diabetes mellitus. And as with most of those millions, very few persons other than the person affected even know she has it. Every day since she was fifteen, Liann has injected herself with insulin and had good control of her blood sugar; she has a college degree in library science and works full-time as a librarian in a university. Recently at age forty, Liann began to experience complications of long-standing diabetes. Her doctor told her that her blood tests showed the beginning of kidney failure. What would she do if her kidneys failed and she required kidney dialysis? How could she keep up her job at the library if she had to take time off several days a week for dialysis treatments?

Liann does have to plan for the future in terms of the time commitment necessary for treatment and how this time will cut into her work day. If she does need dialysis, this could take many hours a week and involve several days a week. Having to either leave work during the day or miss work altogether disrupts schedules and affects job performance. In addition, when treatments such as dialysis or chemotherapy for cancer treatment cause nausea or other discomforts, it may be necessary to go home and not return to work at all. Physiotherapy treatments in cystic fibrosis and other lung diseases may need to be repeated several times during the day; in these instances, a normal nine-to-five work schedule is impossible to adhere to.

In serious illnesses like these, there is no getting around the extensive treatments required. However, one almost always has some options or alternatives in the timing or type of the treatment. For example, if dialysis is necessary, arrangements can be made for the treatments to be carried out in a center near the home or place of work. There are different types of dialysis, peritoneal and hemodialysis. New types of peritoneal dialysis—for those who are amenable to this—can be done by the patient himself while he works, and require no time away from work. Many patients can even do their own hemodialysis at home on off-work hours. Even for those who must be dialyzed at centers, many centers run two or three schedules so that most of the treatment can be completed outside of normal work hours. The same is true of chemotherapy centers where drugs can be received, for example, as an outpatient in the evening.

What is necessary for people who might require this sort of extensive and time-consuming treatment is to plan ahead so that as little disruption as possible occurs both in their work and personal lives. This planning should be done by first talking in detail with one's physician, specialist, or nurse specialist, who will be administering or supervising treatments, and exploring all options.

The next step is to talk to the boss. More often than not, the employer will be supportive, especially of trusted and reliable employees. At any rate, absences from work will become obvious soon enough, and it is better for this to be discussed with the employer before rather than after the fact. If work schedules need to be rearranged, giving the boss (and the employee) some time to work this out and make adjustments in responsibilities is important. Bosses can even help make time available and take unnecessary pressure off while the treatments are going on. Bosses can be supportive and act as a buffer during these stressful times. Treatments such as chemotherapy or dialysis can cause discomfort, so that on some treatment days going back to work might be difficult. Having a boss's cooperation at these times can make it much easier. Trying to go it alone without the boss's knowledge can increase your stress remarkably and cause misunderstandings and poor evaluations when you have unavoidable but unexcused absences.

Planning ahead with one's physician so that the limitations and treatment options are clear, talking with one's boss about scheduling changes, and looking into resources and aids to overcome new disabilities as the result of the illness, can permit one to remain working for many years beyond the appearance of serious complications. Working as long as possible helps one to feel independent and functioning. It is an important way to avoid social isolation as well.

However, while it is one thing to work out a schedule, it is another to feel energetic enough to manage work and treatment.

Treatment side effects, as well as emotional reactions to these physical problems, can make it hard to keep functioning and going to work each day. It may be helpful to also speak with professionals or other persons dealing with the same illnesses and treatments to help yourself cope with the losses and the fears and sadness they bring.

Liann's planning should also include the possibility of job retraining so that, if necessary, she might work more at home, especially if she does her treatments at home and can work while doing them. Maybe she could get some computer equipment at home that would tie in with her workplace and open up other options to continue her work.

♦ The first step toward a good and positive adjustment—and one that can eliminate unnecessary, further emotional pain—is the early recognition of certain work limitations and an early, honest appraisal of one's capabilities.

♦ Before making a decision to give up a job, have a frank discussion with the boss. Alternatives like decreasing hours or days, or taking on less physically demanding work, are frequently possible.

♦ Premature retirement, unless forced by the degree of physical limitations or the employer, should not be encouraged.

♦ Planning for the future is critical. Investigate all possible financial resources.

♦ Volunteering can be a very rewarding contribution to society. Working for money is not the only way to feel productive.

♦ Giving the ill or disabled person jobs around the house, asking his/her opinion, and expressing concern over withdrawal from family affairs, are ways to let the ill or disabled person know that he/she is important.

♦ Making two sets of plans, one which anticipates the possibility of further disabling changes as the illness progresses, leads to less disappointment and surprises later.

- When treatments such as chemotherapy or dialysis are necessary, it is possible to plan ahead and find alternative treatments which disrupt work hours as little as possible.

- Planning ahead with one's physician so that the limitations and treatment options are clear, talking with one's boss about scheduling changes and job options, looking into aids and resources to overcome current disabilities and future ones if they occur, can permit one to remain working for many years.

- Discussing with the family openly and honestly the necessary modifications in life-style that may now be necessary can be very helpful. Don't be embarrassed or guilty about the changes you are asking the family to make. Family members may surprise you and be able to volunteer ways that they can help to make things easier.

CHAPTER 15

Meeting Family Social Responsibilities

The positions each of us occupies within our family and community are many faceted. As a father and husband, a man might be expected to be the major income earner, but he might also be expected to set standards for intrafamily relationships, settle disputes, make financial and social decisions, mete out discipline, and play some part in major activities and milestones. Another set of parallel expectations might exist for a woman.

The demands of an illness on all family members and the actual physical impact on the affected person often interferes with his/her ability to fulfill the expected roles. Even when family members recognize that the illness is responsible for one not being able to fulfill his expected role, it sometimes is difficult to avoid resentment and even grief at the loss. With a bit of creativity, family activities can be modified so that the ill person can have a reduced commitment, yet still satisfy his responsibility in the eyes of the family and himself and thereby maintain dignity and self-esteem. The Marty (stroke) and Mary (cancer) vignettes illustrate problems that can occur when parents are ill and children reach life milestones in which the parents normally play a large part. Irwin (lung disease) illustrates how some extended family members can lose their place in the family because of illness; and finally, the case of Jim (retinitis pigmentosa) illustrates a young family in which the father cannot participate in the children's normal day-to-day activities of growing up. The discussion offers approaches to fulfilling family obligations, and centers on how difficulties in meeting these obligations can be dealt with.

Marty

◆ Marty was very uneasy about his upcoming high school graduation. It should have been the first big milestone of his life, but inside his feelings were in turmoil. Deep down he knew this confusion was because of his dad. His dad was really proud of him and would want to be there, but what a hassle that would be! Dad had had a stroke two years ago, and the once powerful and almost intimidating person was confined to a wheelchair. His mind was intact, alright, but his speech was impaired, and sometimes saliva drooled out of his mouth. Marty was not sure he could bear to have his father there, yet in a way he wanted him there more than anything.

This dilemma is very common. Marty's dad is likely having some of the very same feelings. He certainly does not want to be an embarrassment to his son, and since parents are very perceptive about how their children feel about a disability like this, he is likely quite aware of Marty's inner ambivalence.

Teenagers often worry excessively about what their friends will think of them because of their parent's illness and physical changes. They worry about being pitied or being seen as different. It is very important to overcome these feelings in a situation like that discussed. It will be the only time Marty graduates; if his father misses it, there will be no chance to replay it. Ten years in the future, what will be important to Marty will be very different. Marty will not even remember that he worried about his peers' reactions, but he will remember and be thankful that his father was able to attend his graduation.

Although it is normal to feel embarrassed, this should not be translated into meaning the father should be excluded. In fact, it makes it much easier if it is not a negotiable subject. This can be handled quite easily by the father taking the initiative and taking Marty aside and saying, "Look, son, I know you feel kind of singled out by having a dad with a disability, and I know it can be embarrassing and you might hear some nasty remarks, but I am really proud of you and I really want to be a part of your graduation."

Marty, as other children, most likely feels anxious about how his father will be seen as well as guilty about not wanting him to attend his graduation. His dad can respect these feelings without opting not to go to the graduation; Marty's father can feel good about a decision to attend if he realizes Marty's relative youth and oversensitivity to the pressure of his peers, and if he realizes how much Marty will regret not having had his father there as he matures.

Learning to accept the changes that injury and illness bring is the whole family's job. Teenage years are difficult even without illness. It is important to share with Marty and other children the full nature of his dad's illness. If Marty were involved early in discussions with health professionals, he would understand what is happening and have a good sense about what his dad can and cannot do. Children frequently go through periods of feeling angry and sad. Sometimes embarrassment is covering up these painful feelings and is the expression of their anger, fear, and grief. The most important thing is not to change or alter attending once-in-a-lifetime events. A child marries and graduates only once, and it is very important to celebrate these events.

One of the lessons of life that Marty's dad is showing his son is that adversity in life can be overcome and that despite illness and disability, participation in family and life events can go on. In addition, by allowing their participation in family problems, by learning to talk openly with them about the illness, and by assisting them in planning ways that the ill person can participate in social events, children are helped to become caring, mature adults.

It is also useful to remember that friends rarely react as negatively as we predict they might. Our problems are not on the minds of other people as much as we think they are. Most people are more concerned with their own problems. After living with a person with these problems, one quickly learns that the person has not changed at all and the qualities of a parent whom we love and are proud of, and that our friends respond to, are still there and have not changed. It is also useful to remember that almost every family has experienced some sort of medical problem or crisis, so that being in that situation is probably not so different after all.

◆ Marty's dad, Dale, was worried about the upcoming graduation as well, but his concerns were somewhat different. He had come to terms with the limitations of his stroke and the occasional stares of strangers. What he did not like was being left alone in his wheelchair, or having people feel compelled to complete sentences for him because of the speech limitations left by the stroke. He also worried that Marty might be too embarrassed by his appearance and might ignore him at the ceremony that he wanted very much to attend. If that happened, it would be almost too much to bear.

Let us reiterate that it is a common and irrevocable mistake to think that one should spare the child embarrassment and stay home. The ill person, through feelings of hurt, embarrassment, or self-pity, must not allow the son's immature attitude to rule the day. The decision must be taken out of the hands of the child. Often a child, who is very much influenced by peer pressure but also secretly wants his parent there, will actually be glad for this to happen. It allows him to have his father at the ceremony but also allows him, in interactions with his peers to pass the blame for the attendance onto his father.

Communication between the parent and child about why it has been decided that the parent will attend a life event is critical. It is also necessary that the parent be sensitive to and understanding of the child's feelings. Patience can be a great virtue.

While taking a firm stand and carrying through with it in this situation is nearly always the best solution, we do not pretend that it is easy. Parents will have conflicting feelings about this if the decision is not totally harmonious, but these feelings will fade in time and the person will be very glad he attended the event. Communication far in advance of family social events can alleviate many concerns before they really become issues, and necessary modifications of the events can be made so that everyone feels wanted and as comfortable as possible. The initiative is best taken by the ill person who can give suggestions that will optimize the experience of everyone.

When a child is particularly distressed about a decision that has been made, or if he feels his rights have been squashed, a compromise might be offered that would not affect the main event. For example, if Marty would like to go off with his friends after the ceremony rather than attend a family gathering, that may be a good compromise.

Far in advance of events like a graduation or a wedding, the family must have a meeting to plan the event. Talking together about what each person needs to feel comfortable at the event allows the family to formulate a good plan of action. For example, Marty's mother will take his father to the event; having arrived, Marty, who has picked up his girlfriend and is waiting at the hall, will assist his mother in getting his dad out of the car and into the chair, etc. Once a plan for the entire event is worked out that satisfies all parties' concerns, Marty will not worry that he will not get to spend time with his friends, and Dale will not need to worry that he will be abandoned. If he can attend and see his son's graduation, other things he needs from his son can wait till he has reached a better level of maturity. Dale's respect for his son's feelings will be a model for his son to respect his feelings.

An important side benefit of such an approach to organizing a milestone event is that Marty and his friends learn that people with disabilities are not lepers and are not to be forgotten. Learning how much people can do despite the illness, learning patience when someone has difficulty speaking, learning not to feel so uncomfortable around disease and illness, can help each person accept more quickly the life events that happen to them. If Marty's dad respects himself, he will be respected by Marty.

◆ As the graduation day approached, Dale realized there were other more practical problems to contend with as well. The school had twenty steps, and there was no easy way to get the wheelchair up them. Furthermore, a dinner was to be served for the parents, and Dale knew he would not be able to eat without soiling his clothes unless someone helped him. And that could be embarrassing.

Some illnesses, or physical deficits and limitations, require that special arrangements must be considered and made in advance. Calling on the extended family again can be very helpful. Other family members such as cousins, aunts and uncles, or even good friends can be solicited to lend a hand. If asked in advance, these persons usually are more than willing to help.

Sometimes young, strong teenagers are perfect people to help. Teenagers can be demanding and harsh, but they can also be very sensitive and humane. If Marty were strong and secure enough to ask some of his friends to help, he might find that their attitude about his father was far different than he imagined. More than likely, they would be willing not only to help get his dad to the graduation but may use this as an opportunity to talk to Marty about his dad and express some of their concern for him and his dad. Including of friends in activities makes them feel wanted and relieves a lot of unspoken tension. It is a way for the ill or disabled family member to maintain social connections and avoid social isolation.

But if Marty is too embarrassed to ask his friends, then family members need to be included and used to help with the accessibility issues. Dale's wife can help him with the dinner. He can get specially designed forks to help with eating so that it is easier to pick up food and not drop it. Also, there is the option of not eating much dinner but attending the dinner. It is not necessary to eat at all affairs if one finds it very difficult or embarrassing to try. What is important is to do what feels comfortable. Attending the functions is the most important part of it as well as being included in the pictures and having memories and experiences to talk about later. It feels like a normal thing to do as well, and brings back the experience of doing things as a family again. It is impossible to pretend that no changes have taken place and foolhardy not to make advance preparations for the events. Special equipment, aids, or even extra people to help, all must be reserved in advance. Needless to say, without this type of proper planning, attending the event can become a disaster and a very big disappointment for everyone.

Mary

◆ Mary was very pleased that her daughter Joann had decided to marry her longtime boyfriend Ed. Two years ago she would have relished the role of mother of the bride, but now with a recent and devastating diagnosis of breast cancer, she was not sure she was quite up to it. Nevertheless, she felt obligated to fulfill her duty. After a month of planning, meeting with caterers, and non-stop organizing, Mary was beat! The old, boundless energy was gone; and she found that the chemotherapy treatments she was taking made her feel even weaker. She had come to wish that Joann and Ed would elope.

Mary and the family may be thinking that Mary's total control of the preparations will help her overcome the emotional effects of cancer. However, it may be that even without the cancer chemotherapy, which does take a lot out of a person, Mary should have more help with the planning. Feeling obligated to fulfill her duty probably was a personality trait of Mary's before she was slowed down by illness. Likely, people took advantage of her willingness to do things even then.

Mary needs to assert herself a bit more and make it clear that the job is too much for her. She need not feel guilty about this; it is not one person's—even a well person's—obligation to take on everything. Mary must take the initiative and tell her daughter that she cannot do it by herself. She can suggest instead that she be the foreman. She can organize a mutual effort using her daughter, daughters-in-law, possibly sisters, and others, and delegate the various duties so that no one will be overworked. With so many doing the actual legwork, Mary can act as the coordinator to make sure everyone's efforts mesh and result in the perfect wedding.

Being able to ask for what you need is an important skill for adults to learn. For Mary, trying to plan a whole wedding by herself is in some way denying that she has a life-threatening illness that needs some of her attention. She needs to also take care of herself and acknowledge the current limitations. It is not only acceptable, but also important, to acknowledge limitations and admit that one cannot handle the whole load. In fact, it can be physically harmful and foolhardy to undertake too much under the misconception that it is one's duty.

Generally children and others enjoy working with the parents in planning a wedding. It is a joyous event, and getting everyone involved makes them feel a part of the event. It also is a way that Mary and her daughter can be close and enjoy each other. Elopement is not necessary, just a scaling down and redistribution of duties among family members.

Unfortunately, sometimes the person who is overburdened by the very nature of his/her accommodating personality will fail to recognize that the job is overwhelming or, alternatively, will not want to admit to the impact of the illness on their energy. Then another family member may have to step in and help the ill or disabled person carry the load. This can be done without any conversation which might be too embarrassing for the ill person. A family member who does not wait to be asked to do chores but jumps right in and does them, can efficiently take a large load off Mary.

◆ Mary's sister, Deirdre, had noticed the toll that the wedding preparations were taking on her sister and decided to step in. Though she had a part-time job, she offered to help, and after talking with Joann and Ed, all agreed that a simpler, less time-consuming ceremony would be more appropriate for everyone.

If it is necessary, adjusting the social event is a possible solution. When the ill person does not suggest modifications, someone else in a respected position in the family may be able to revamp that commitment so that it is not so large and difficult, yet the ill person can still feel a part of things and important in the planning of the event.

For example, a father expected to carve and serve Thanksgiving dinner, but unable to because of Parkinson's Disease, can choose who his carving successor may be and advise him as to the best way to carve. He can also choose another role he can fulfill at dinner—like leading grace or proposing the toast—instead if he wishes. Talking about this before it is time to carve the turkey (or whatever the responsibility is) allows the ill person to participate in the change and thus still feel important and involved in the family decisions. If it is left to the moment when the turkey needs to be carved, then it can be an embarrassing moment. There are many little things that each member of a family participates in that we often take for granted until a disability or illness prevents them from being able to do those things. The ill person may recognize this far in advance and worry unduly about his/her inability to perform that function; they may even become depressed or irritable because of the fear that when faced with fulfilling the function, they will fail. It is important not to pretend that nothing has happened but to admit that the changes have occurred, and then to move on and find new ways to help the ill or disabled person maintain an important role in the family event. Since family members may not think of the particular function the ill person will not be able to perform any longer, it is incumbent on the ill person to bring this up in family discussions, well in advance of the event so that alternate plans can be put into action.

◆ Mary felt relieved about the change of plans, but she still felt anxious about the wedding. She had noticed that since the cancer diagnosis, some people seemed to avoid speaking to her, and she was afraid that some of the friends might turn down invitations because of her illness. She also worried that she would become too fatigued with the activities of the reception and dancing and would have to leave early before the guests.

Mary's biggest difficulty is trying to be all that she thinks she should be, as if she is not facing and dealing with a very serious illness. It is very important to acknowledge the new limitations without guilt or denial. The most important thing is that Mary is attending the wedding. She is not missing an important family function because she is afraid that people will avoid her or turn down invitations. She is participating in a once-in-a-lifetime event that she will remember forever and talk about with her grandchildren. She is sharing a moment with her children that draws them closer to each other. It is a happy time in the family and a time to rejoice. Certainly there are enough events in life that bring sadness—like the cancer and stress—that when there is a fun family social activity, it is vital that Mary allow herself to enjoy it and not continually worry about how her illness will mar it.

Some of Mary's concerns reflect the stigmatizing effects of a cancer diagnosis and her concerns about this. People sometimes do turn down invitations because they know someone has cancer. Such an action would almost certainly hurt unduly the suffering person and add to her burden of grief and anger. These people could hardly be called real friends and would not likely have been good guests.

It is highly unlikely that anyone would notice if Mary left early, or if she danced or not. Most people would be happy to see her there enjoying the event, regardless of how long she stays. How much Mary participates depends on how well she is feeling. People understand limitations, even if they do not always know what to say in response to illness or disability, and that can always be the reason for leaving early or refusing a dance. Mary has to do what is best for her health and not what she sees as the expectations of others. She has to meet her own needs as well as work with her family to meet their needs.

Irwin

◆ Joann's great uncle Irwin had advanced lung disease. She loved him dearly but thought that if she invited him to her wedding, which was small, he would feel obligated to come. And she knew that just walking a few feet made him short of breath; it would be simply too stressful for him. So she did not send an invitation. Irwin was deeply hurt.

People still have feelings even though illness is limiting their life-styles; they need to be remembered and not left out of the family events. Even if they cannot come, they are still part of the family and deserve recognition as such. Perhaps, under the surface, Joann has mixed feelings about his attending the wedding in the first place. It can be sad to see someone you love deteriorating.

The most common mistake is to think it is better to spare the ill or disabled person the embarrassment of having to turn you down or to face the limitations that their injury or illness now imposes on them. This takes all sense of control and sense of self-worth from the ill person. Out of her good intentions not to hurt Irwin's feelings, Joann made a unilateral decision and took choice away from him. He is not allowed to choose whether or not to come; you, in effect, are saying that you know what he can and cannot do better than he does. Unintentionally you are removing from him a role that was once very important.

If Irwin decides that he cannot attend, that is a far better way for him to be excluded. Not issuing an invitation may cause ill feelings that could last for years. If another family member volunteers feelings that the ill or disabled person might not want to attend, or that it might be too much trouble for him/her to attend, it is important to find out what is behind these feelings. Did the ill person express such feelings to the family member? Or is the opinion expressed simply that of the family member?

Without too much trouble, special arrangements can usually be made. For example, Irwin could have extra oxygen arranged and have an attendant accompany him so that he can have extra help walking, if necessary, or a companion if he has to leave the party for intervals to rest. It is important to make it clear to the ill or disabled person that you want him to attend, and then offer to find ways to help him do it. Nothing speaks louder than actions. Seeing that the necessary cot is brought in to the lounge in case Irwin gets tired and needs to lie down, or that the oxygen tanks are ordered for him, truly lets him know that he is wanted.

Jim

◆ When he was twenty-eight, Jim began to lose his eyesight from a hereditary disease called retinitis pigmentosa. He had known that he might develop this because his uncle had had it, and so he had chosen a sales career in which most of his work could be done via telephone and tape recorder and was not dependent on his eyesight. Even though he had planned for an uncertain future, he had not anticipated the problems that were developing with his son, James Jr., age ten. James had always had a close relationship with his father, but lately he was becoming moody and uncommunicative and would not respond to Jim's inquiries about what was bothering him. Finally, one night after one more attempt to discern the problem, James said, "Nobody else's mother drives them to hockey practice or Boy Scouts."

James needs to understand that his father cannot influence the changes that are happening in him, and the family will need to adapt to the changes. He will understand better about this, and why his father is not driving him, if he understands better what is happening to his father. He will also be less frightened and insecure. The illness his father is trying to cope with needs to be explained to James simply, without the implication at this point in time, that it is hereditary. For example, Jim can say to James: "James, I would like to tell you what is happening to my eyes. Would you like to know why I don't drive you anymore? It is unfortunate, but I am having more and more trouble seeing because of a problem in my eyes. The doctor has told me that it can't get better, so I have to make changes in the way I do things. You have seen the new equipment I have bought for my work so that I don't need to use my eyes so much. While I am happy to find ways to keep working, I am very sad about other things I have to give up because of my bad eyes. One of them is driving you to your hockey games. Because my eyes are not so good any more, I can't drive. However, I still hope we can do things together. OK? Do you have any questions about my eyes?"

This will also enable James to know what to say to his friends if they ask him why his father is not driving him, as this is something which sets him apart from them. James's father should sit down with him and work out a statement that James can tell the friends that ask about his father.

Participating in the care of an ill parent gives a child a sense of responsibility. Identifying ways in which James can help his father is important. In addition to learning about the limitations of his father's illness, James undoubtedly will think of ways that he can

238   BUILDING A NEW DREAM

be with his father and his father can participate in the things that are important to him. They can plan together the ways his father can contribute in other aspects of his life. James Jr. may need to express his sadness about what has happened to his dad. It does little good to shield a child and not give him an opportunity to express his feelings, ask questions, and plan ways to be together. A child does not realize unless it is pointed out to him that he is experiencing feelings of loss and bewilderment.

◆ When Jim recognized James Jr.'s feeling of loss, he realized that so much time had been devoted to coping with his visual deficits that he had not only neglected James Jr., but in doing so, had shifted extra burdens onto his wife. He set aside special times every week when he and his son could spend time alone together in a variety of activities.

It is important to remember that children have a life apart from the family that does not include illness. It is important to spend time with James Jr. and his friends in fun ways. Focus on what is possible instead of what is not possible. The more time that is spent doing activities that are possible rather than talking about what cannot be done, the less frequently anyone feels left out or even as aware of the limitations of the illness or disability. If James Jr. feels he is getting enough love and attention, he will be able to modify his expectations of his father and find ways to accommodate the father's limitations in his time alone with him and with his friends. Open communication about things that can and cannot be done, as well as feelings about these limitations, permits good relationships and accommodation to the changes imposed by illness or disability. Jim can invite James to talk about the things they can do together. What are James's suggestions? He can also ask him about his feelings about the changes in their relationship by simply inquiring about those activities he used to do with James before his loss of eyesight prevented it. For example, Jim can be playing cards with James. While they are playing, he can ask James, "How are the trips to the hockey games these days? Is Mom a decent driver?" James can still feel like dad's buddy in these new ways.

◆ When illness or disability saps your strength and turns minor everyday chores into time-consuming projects, it is difficult to find the time and energy to participate in family events.

◆ Children and family members must be careful to put aside feelings of embarrassment, and instead, encourage the disabled or ill person and assist him/her in participating in family activities. Including the disabled or ill person prevents him/her from falling out of the family matrix and becoming isolated.

◆ When a disabled person is part of a family event, it is very important to make detailed plans in advance. Make sure that proper access, special equipment, and other necessary special preparations are worked out well in advance. This will make the event enjoyable for everyone.

◆ Parents are often expected to make the preparations for events like marriages and graduations. When a parent is ill, he or she can still be a part of the planning, but both the parent and child(ren) must recognize that the burden of the workload must be shifted to someone else.

◆ When an ill relative no longer can participate in family activities in his/her usual role, the family must find new ways to include him/her.

◆ Young children are aware of illness in a parent and need to talk about it. They need to be reassured that it was not caused by their misbehavior, and that it is not catching. Allowing them to share in the person's care without giving them excessive responsibility, makes children feel important and involved.

CHAPTER 16

Fighting Social Isolation

When a family begins to cope with a newly diagnosed chronic illness, social activities are often the furthest thing from their minds. Thus, the stage is set early in an illness for a gradual withdrawal from the social activities and groups that could be a very positive support for the ill person and the family.

Preoccupation with the medical problem, as well as a reluctance to have others know about the illness, may result in the family setting up barriers to interaction with their usual social circles. While some may find it difficult to deal with illness in a friend, this type of reaction is usually much less prevalent than it is perceived to be by the affected family. In fact, early social withdrawal is hard to correct later on when friendships have waned and the illness is more physically taxing. It also becomes more difficult for an ill person to make the efforts required to establish new friendships. The loneliness and isolation for the whole family can be devastating on the family relationships, because our sense of self and our place in society, as well as the family's role in the community, depends on social interactions.

Support from extended family members and others in the community can be very helpful in the adjustment and coping process. Mel and Eileen, in this chapter, address the social stresses of a near-retirement couple who find themselves coping first with a mental, then a physical disability. A younger couple with children, Tracy and Mac, face somewhat different social barriers when one of them falls ill. The vignettes about Madelyn and Leo illustrate approaches to some of the problems that single persons dealing with physical deformity might encounter. Finally, the vignettes about Raymond and Stephanie address the special issues related to AIDS and to an adolescent recovering from cancer and chemotherapy treatment. Hopefully, these vignettes will help you recognize early pitfalls leading to social isolation, and suggest to you ways of maintaining social contact even though your participation as a person or family may have to be modified somewhat.

Mel and Eileen

◆ Eileen's Alzheimer's Disease arrived painfully early at age fifty-five; nevertheless, Mel faithfully cared for her as her memory faded. He continued an active life-style both by working full-time and by playing tennis regularly with several of his buddies. Unfortunately, the activities that he and Eileen had enjoyed together seemed to be falling by the wayside; no longer did they play bridge together because her concentration was failing, nor did they visit the country club as often. People, it seemed to Mel, avoided them at the club, as it was becoming difficult to have relevant conversations with Eileen, and he felt somehow embarrassed by this. He felt more comfortable hiring an attendant to stay with Eileen while he went out alone.

Caring for an ill or disabled person when there is a gradual deterioration, is very demanding and tiring. The daily routine of care; the dependency, anxiety, and depression felt or expressed by the ill or disabled person; personality changes; and the increased forgetfulness of dementing illnesses emotionally exhaust the caretaker. While it is important for the caretaker to have activities, and family or private help to gain a respite (see Chapter 10: Preventing Emotional Exhaustion), it is also important to monitor whether or not the extent to which the family members pursue their own interests is not fostering social isolation for the ill person.

It is surprising how much more frequently, after the symptoms of a gradually debilitating and obvious disease like multiple sclerosis, Parkinson's Disease, or Huntington's Disease worsen, that the family will go to activities without the ill person. The family members may believe that the embarrassment they feel is also felt by the ill person and that by leaving them behind, they are relieving them of unnecessary embarrassment and hurt. This also enables the ill or disabled person, if they are feeling freakish, to avoid the discomfort of being different.

Persons with dementing illness, more so than other illnesses, may also develop behaviors that are considered socially unacceptable and which become difficult to manage both in the home and especially in the community. Mel is experiencing some of the social consequences of these changes. A typical behavior of a person with a dementing illness is that he/she will ask the same question over and over, or repeat a story again and again. Socially, this can be embarrassing and annoying for family members. Not only are peoples' reactions of annoyance, anger, and abandonment of the person with the dementing illness, confusing and hurtful for him/her, but it is also hurtful for family members. It is difficult to accept that a person who was once socially very skilled, had many friends, and was invited to many parties would now say embarrassing things to good friends, forget who people were, and repeat himself so much that being with him becomes so uncomfortable that former friends no longer want to be around him. Denial that the dementia is happening and a wish that the ill person would be himself again are common responses.

Leaving such a person home while they participate in social activities, permits the family not to have to deal with their own feelings—usually of emotional pain, fear, grief, and sadness. Not uncommonly, the person suffering from loss of memory and confusion will isolate himself so that he/she doesn't have to feel different, hurt, or socially inept.

Another reaction of family members toward a person suffering dementing illness is anger directed at the person. Close relatives, spouses, and siblings can become expressively angry at the ill person. They want him/her to just stop odd behaviors, and they imply that the person could if he/she really wanted to. It is important for the family to understand that the ill person has no control over the behavior, that it is not deliberate or hostile behavior, and that he/she is probably as embarrassed by it as the relatives are.

Further, such persons cannot stop themselves. Anger at them does not help or change anything; it simply results in frustration. Anger does help the family member deny the permanent changes occurring in a loved family member, and masks the fear and sadness this brings.

If anger doesn't help, what might help? To avoid social isolation, it is very important for the ill or disabled person to remain involved and to participate at family and social functions. It is very important for ill and disabled persons to remain as active and as social as possible. The person's family can foster postive adjustment to the life changes caused by the illness by encouraging the afflicted family member to continue socializing. For example, when we include someone at a party, who has been confined to a wheelchair as a result of a progressive physical illness, who has dementing illness, who has a diagnosis of terminal cancer, we are telling these people nonverbally, by the invitation, that we still want to be friends and that we can handle the changes which have happened to them without feeling unduly uncomfortable. When extended family and friends plan functions in accessible places, they don't have to say they want the ill or disabled person there. It is obvious. Sometimes it is easier and very effective to express caring nonverbally. Picnics, walks, movies, and other community events are possible activities for the family.

In order to help close friends adapt to the person's disability, they should be taken into your confidence and told about the problem, be it physical or mental, and the changes to expect. Friends often need to be reassured that their presence is still wanted and needed. Sometimes they have to be told how to be helpful and reassured about what to talk about with the ill/disabled person.

Embarrassment about their continuing health in the face of their friend's illness (why were they spared?) and the anxiety about illness in general can cause certain friends to disappear. But those friends who can cope with their feelings about loss and their own vulnerability to illness will remain caring and helpful if the family allows them to do so. These friendships can be made more enduring. This can be done, for example, by inviting people over, or eating out with friends who understand the problems and are not embarrassed by physical debility or by the behaviors of persons suffering from dementing illness. But continued contact—which you, the family of the ill person, often must initiate—must be maintained, or all the friends will fall by the wayside. These relationships, like any others, require ongoing attention and work.

Finally, to help prevent social isolation, family members must talk about the fears associated with loss of self-esteem and prestige. These same feelings can be shared with close friends and other supportive family members. In addition, the family unit may need to deal with their own grief and loss. Progressive illnesses and disabilities resulting from worsening illnesses create great stress for the family. If the family is having a lot of trouble with unexpressed feelings, it is helpful to talk with the doctor, social worker, or psychologist about their reaction to the changes and behavior in the person with a dementing or progressive illness.

◆ About two years after the onset of Eileen's illness, Mel noticed something particularly distressing. He was having a hard time keeping up with his pals at tennis. He was becoming more and more short of breath and found it difficult to finish a game. The problem was diagnosed as emphysema by his doctor. In the next year, he was forced to give up tennis. At first he continued to go to the club every Saturday to socialize with the guys, but it did not take a genius to realize that they were spending less and less time with him. Things became even tougher when Mel had to start using supplemental oxygen supplied by a little tank he carried with him, because now the guys could no longer smoke around him. One day he found that they had organized a social function and had not invited him.

With debilitating physical as well as mental problems, those one thought were close and caring friends suddenly do not call anymore. It is embarrassing, and it hurts. It also is difficult for you to approach them, because you fear—often correctly—that you will be rejected. A phone call may result in polite conversation about how busy they are, but not in arranging a time to be together. This hurts, is humiliating, and makes the ill person angry and uncomfortable.

In Mel's case, not being able to smoke any more does not seem like a reason not to be included, especially if his friends want to be with him. For them, however, it is a convenient excuse to avoid feeling uncomfortable. We have many cultural taboos in our society, centered around illness. Being ill makes one different and sets one apart from the accepted norm. It is not acceptable to have a weakness like illness, and being around someone who has succumbed to this reminds us of our own vulnerability and mortality. Therefore, asking someone to interact with an ill person is, in a sense, asking them to associate with someone who is culturally unacceptable. Many people simply do not know what to say to or how to act around someone who is ill or disabled; we are never taught how to interact with people who are ill. We are unsure whether it is the same or different from how we interact with the mainstream "well" population. This discomfort about what to say and how to behave causes us to avoid ill or disabled persons.

It is very important for the ill or disabled person to recognize that he is not responsible for how the people around him feel and act. Their withdrawal is a function of who those people are, and not who the ill person is. Though it will undoubtedly hurt and be a reminder of the consequences of illness and disability, he must recognize that. There will be friends who will not be frightened and will remain helpful and caring. These friendships have to be cultivated; it is just as easy for well friends to feel hurt and neglected by their suffering buddy if they have been abandoned by him and not allowed to share his suffering and companionship. It is the responsibility of the ill person and the family not to become totally consumed by the illness, to the exclusion of their true friends. They must continue to nurture relationships with people who remain friends, despite the anger about those who could not.

Close and enduring friends want to share important parts of your life with you and be there to comfort you when necessary. To allow them to do this, you must bring up your illness or disability in conversations with them. Both you and they know that this has happened to you; not acknowledging that is like having another person in the room whom you are both ignoring. Now, is that an uncomfortable feeling?! Help make friends comfortable by talking openly about things in a futuristic and optimistic way without complaining and without despair.

In speaking about your illness or disability, however, it is important that you not dwell on how unfortunate you are. Everyone is sorry that this happened to you, but what can they do about it? Dwelling on your bad luck makes them feel as if you somehow expect them to make it go away. Besides, it is very difficult to stay around a constantly complaining person for very long. When friends begin to feel depressed or feel that nothing they say will help, they will avoid those feelings by avoiding the ill or disabled person. It is also important not to berate friends or family members for not calling more often, or to instantly report to them how terrible things have been. They know you have had a tough time; being with them might make you feel better. Being socially active and participating in family and community activities gives the ill or disabled something other than themselves or their physical problems to think about and to talk about.

◆ As if the problems of isolation facing Mel and Eileen were not bad enough, they soon felt that even their daughter, Ellen, had abandoned them. To some extent, this was true. Ellen had always thought of her parents as invincible; now the infirmities of advancing age were all too apparent. While she had made a point of bringing the grandchildren to visit or having her folks over for dinner at least once a week, she now seemed to find excuses not to see them. Deep inside she had a nagging sense of guilt about this. Even worse, she was beginning to feel uncomfortable around her parents, especially her mother who increasingly seemed more like a child.

It is very hard to watch people whom we have respected and looked to for advice and as role models, become weak and unable to be in charge. When the personality changes, as in Eileen's case, it is almost as if the person we knew has died, yet she has not. Her body is still there, and she still looks the same, but the person is a stranger. We watch helplessly as the person becomes less and less familiar; withdrawal and anger follow. It is common to feel embarrassment, but this really is usually another way of expressing guilt and sadness. It is a sad time, a time for mourning the losses and changes. When family members age, it is also a reminder that we are aging. The sense of time passing sometimes is felt for the first time, and this also elicits feelings of pain and sadness. It is important to realize, though not very comforting, that you are not going to be able to make the disease go away. There is no miracle cure. It is just as important to recognize that you did not cause the illness, and you did nothing to bring it into your life or the suffering person's life. In some families, it is possible to share some of these feelings with the ill person and the caretaker. If that's possible, it is a good way to feel better and to feel closer to one another. After taking some time to grieve, Ellen should be able to spend more time with her mother. She may find this difficult at times, when her mother forgets things and seems confused, but whatever they can share together now, she will have as memories after her mother's death.

Frequently, adult children are fearful that spending time with their family means giving up their freedom and time totally to care for the disabled or ill parent. Ellen can help her father and mother avoid isolation without increased dependency on her by helping them locate church-run groups, Alzheimer support groups for herself and her father, and by contacting the American Lung Association for groups and activities for her father. She can also call on other family members to help relieve her father and enable him to get out of the house. Relatives can take turns taking care of some of the housekeeping duties which now, with his lung disease, can be too difficult for Mel. Ellen could also help her father by running errands, or making business calls related to her mother's illness, for him. It is possible to be very helpful by calling in two or three times a week to see if there is anything you can do. Just calling to say hello sometimes breaks the isolation the caretaker can be feeling. As Eileen's condition worsens, it may become necessary for the family to meet to discuss possible home-care options and nursing homes. This will require Ellen and her father to be able to communicate so that they can make plans that are the best economically and emotionally for everyone. If she can talk openly with her father, they can plan together better and support each other more. The first step is usually the hardest. Ellen can tell her father that she knows how hard it must be for him, because it is hard for her to see her mother deteriorate. This can then lead to an open conversation about how each of them is managing the changes. It is in these various ways that Ellen can be an enormous help, and manage her feelings about what has happened to her parents.

◆ Mel was not a person to sit around and become depressed. One of Mel and Eileen's really trusted friends from early in their marriage, was Eileen's brother, Joe. Mel turned to Joe now for companionship. Joe seemed to accept both his sister's illness and Mel's limitations without embarrassment or uneasiness. Joe, who had always favored more sedentary diversions, soon had Mel playing croquet, shuffleboard, and chess. Eileen could participate in many of these activities as well.

Being active with other people is the most important way to avoid feelings of despair and loneliness. Seeking out family members and friends who are not uneasy and embarrassed with illness or disability, is to take advantage of the opportunity for social activity and social companionship. Concentrating on the friends and family members who cannot feel comfortable only results in sustained feelings of self-pity and despair. There are people who are willing to be a part of one's life, and there are activities which are appropriate for participation by ill and disabled persons. The person will have to address his/her limitations and may have to change interests a bit, however all but the very terminally ill can find some type of activity in which they can participate.

◆ Joe disliked cold weather, and every winter he traveled to Central America for a month or two. This year he invited Mel and Eileen to join him. Mel very much wanted to go, as the cold weather adversely affected his breathing. At the same time, he was very apprehensive. He wondered if he could get oxygen in Central America, and if he would need more because the altitude is greater. What would he do if he became sick? Could they take care of him down there, or what arrangements would have to be made to get back in a hurry. He wondered if he could get oxygen on the plane.

Travel is a wonderful way to be entertained and to get away from the routines and sameness of everyday life. If traveling was a part of one's life before illness or disability, it can be part of one's life again. It may even be something new to try that a person always wanted to do but never could seem to find the time for! And, although certain hotels and cities may be out of consideration, there are many places in the world that are accessible and provide necessary and good medical back-up. For Eileen, the stimulation of travel, especially if it is to places she has frequently gone to and loved, can help her feel active again and not so apathetic.

It is a necessary component of travel after an injury, physical illness, or long-term illness, to plan all details in advance. Being forced to think about travel plans helps an ill or disabled person to feel that there is something for him/her to do that needs to be done. For paralyzed persons or the wheelchair bound, it is important to make prior arrangements, such as finding nurses or aides who can assist the family at the vacation spot. There are travel agents who specialize in arrangements for the disabled or ill person. They can make all kinds of necessary arrangements ahead of time, including letting the airlines know that you are coming, and arranging for accessible accommodations. If necessary, when notified in advance, airlines will provide supplemental oxygen to patients with advanced lung disease, for example. If there is a need to rent a van, that too can be arranged ahead of time. Supplies that are too big to bring can be rented. Finding and locating appropriate hospital facilities and physicians for hemodialysis, regular blood work, or to locate more oxygen, can be done ahead of time with the help of your physician and his office. An organization that can assist with arrangements for disabled travelers is the Society for the Advancement of Travel for the Handicapped. A helpful guide is *Frommer's Guide for the Disabled Traveler,* by Frances Barish, published by Simon and Schuster, Inc.

It can feel like a lot of work and extra money to travel after an illness or disability, because it is now no longer possible to just hop on a plane and go. However, being able to take advantage of travel by air, sea, or car, provides family recreation, provides continued family interaction and memories, and provides entertainment, social interaction, and a sense that life has not changed that much after all. Especially if there are young children in the family, the feeling that you are doing some of the things you would have done if injury or illness had not struck, is a positive feeling that results in more optimistic and hopeful feelings about the future. The more independent and active one is, the less possibility there is of becoming depressed.

Tracy and Mac

◆ Tracy and Mac had a storybook marriage and the "perfect" family, a four-year-old son and a two-year-old daughter, when the first signs of Mac's multiple sclerosis surfaced. The initial numbness and tingling in his left leg went away in a few days, but a month later he lost his eyesight for a few days, and things went downhill from there. Within two years, Mac needed a wheelchair to get around. Tracy had had to get a job to support the family, and Tracy's mother took care of the kids. All in all, the family had coped reasonably well with this disastrous illness, but the one thing that had suffered miserably was their social life.

Even after the children were born, Tracy and Mac had managed to see a movie every two weeks or so, and often went to friends' homes or had friends in for dinner. They also had enjoyed a number of sports. Now Tracy was so tired after working all day and spending time with the kids at night, as well as helping in Mac's care, that she hardly had time even to think about her friends. Actually, they hardly called anymore, probably because she usually turned down their invitations. Yet she could not deny that deep inside she was feeling empty and lonely and maybe a bit depressed at the loss of the camaraderie of their friends. Mac was feeling a bit the same, but Tracy seemed so tired and busy all the time that he was reluctant to bring it up. Besides, he was embarrassed and a bit ashamed about his illness and that he was the cause of their loss of friends.

In this case, the ill person and the family contribute to their current feelings of isolation. When friends are continually turned down without alternative suggestions or definite dates set, they are bound to feel that they are intruding or are not wanted anymore. The ill person and family members may fear that they will be the center of attention socially, and that possibility may make them feel uncomfortable. Families in this situation might have a number of fears. They may think that others feel uncomfortable talking to them about everyday things, or that acquaintances feel they have to choose words carefully to avoid offending the couple who can no longer participate in the activities being discussed. The family may even question whether they will know what to talk about with friends after spending so much time and energy focused on the illness and themselves. While one may feel very vulnerable and insecure socially, the worst thing to do is to withdraw from social events. The only thing to do is bite the bullet and make a definite commitment to a social engagement. You and your family may be different, but all of you still need the support and interaction of your social circle. In a sense, the family with illness will have to work a bit harder; the responsibility is on them to make their community of friends and family comfortable around them. It may seem unfair at first to have to do this too, but only the family members know what they can do physically, know how not to place the ill or disabled person in an invalid role, and understand other peoples' discomfort with illness and disability.

Useful tips to facilitate a family's integration back into the community include reassuring friends that they can ask questions and talk about the injury or illness; letting friends know how to be helpful (for example, how to walk with a wheelchair when walking to a table at a restaurant, or how to help get up stairs or put on clothes); readily answering questions about what causes diseases like multiple sclerosis and assuring them that it is not contagious; and volunteering information about the changes in one's life as a result of illness or disability. This lets people know that they are free to say things and ask questions without hurting feelings or treading on unwelcome territory. As people interact with ill and disabled persons more and more, they will become comfortable with their own behavior.

Spouses and the ill person need to maintain their own individual outlets as well as maintaining their family and social relationships. The ill person himself needs to contact friends and invite them over to his home.

Sometimes the combination of the daily demands that result from a family member becoming ill and the existing emotional responses of anxiety, dependency, and depression, leave family members too exhausted to think about continuing activities that once were an important part of family life. This must not be allowed to happen. If the spouse or caretaker is working too hard, then baby-sitters and other forms of home-health care and help from the family needs to be considered. Joining in family outings to the park or to school activities, calling friends for dinner engagements, going to the movies or out to dinner are necessary. These activities all help the family to feel that they are still part of this world and are normal. It is important to feel that the family can have relaxation and entertainment as part of their life. It is energizing for everyone. Feelings like Mac's, that he is responsible for the loss of friends, or the fear that he will be putting yet another responsibility on Tracy's head, can be avoided if plans are made to contact friends and keep a social network.

Madelyn

◆ Madelyn's life had fallen apart since she developed a Bell's Palsy. She woke up one morning and noticed that one side of her face would not move, almost like what she imagined a stroke to be. The doctor said it would improve in a few days, but it did not. Weeks passed and only a small amount of the movement returned. A vivacious and outgoing schoolteacher, Madelyn felt very self-conscious about her change in appearance. She found it painful to talk about the problem with her friends and was embarrassed in front of her classes. Furthermore, her friends seemed to avoid talking to her, and she thought it was because sometimes she was unable to keep bits of saliva from dribbling out of the paralyzed side of her mouth. Social interactions became more and more difficult, and she began to take sick days from work even though she felt fine.

People who have developed severe physical changes (bodily changes, paralysis, disfigurement) due to progressive illnesses like Lou Gehrig's Disease (amyotrophic lateral sclerosis) or stable illnesses like cerebral palsy, or due to a sudden illness or accident which leaves a dysfunction, can experience disturbing responses from friends, relatives, or society in general. This type of response is really based in cultural prejudices that suggest that disabilities are ugly and that people disabled by illness or injury are freaks, unable to participate with normal people in the work force or be able to be loved. The person who is sick, unfortunately, also in the back of his mind harbors many of these same feelings, because he has been raised with the same cultural background.

These stereotypic responses suggest that people with disabilities are sick, helpless, or retarded. Associating with an ill person in some way connects the well person to the illness, and subconsciously he harbors the fear that it is possible he could get sick, disabled, and die. Maybe the disease *is* really infectious, and he will get it. And being sick is bad. This type of superstitious thinking, without basis in fact, as a response to illness is also a cultural legacy.

For some people, other people's illnesses are to be avoided because of the discomfort it causes. An illness with a clearly visible disfigurement as a constant reminder of the affliction, tends to trigger anxiety in persons who are not ill or disabled. Socially isolating the person who creates this anxiety seems to be the best way to avoid it.

When it is hard to speak and be understood, as in Madelyn's case, it can be difficult and uncomfortable to engage in conversation. The discomfort of the conversation for the well person can cause anxiety, and he may walk away or go to some effort to avoid the ill or disabled person.

All human beings are sensitive to reactions, rejections, lack of eye contact, and the failure to be included in activities. This is not unique to those suffering the ravages of illness, disabilities, or physical disfigurement. We are all concerned with how we look. We all worry about what we perceive to be our imperfections and that we will not meet society's standards of beauty, as physical beauty is one of the highly prized attributes in our culture. Being beautiful almost assures, or certainly greatly simplifies, acceptance into the society. Everyone feels some insecurity about his or her physical attributes.

Thus, while it is important for persons experiencing physical changes due to illness or disability to feel that their physical changes are not cause for exclusion from their social groups, it is equally important for their social contacts to feel that way. Or in spite of the person's best efforts, he/she will become socially isolated. Sometimes surgical intervention, like reconstructive surgery after breast removal or grafting after severe burns, can be performed, and this can help with issues related to self-esteem and appearance. And that emotional boost, along with the physical changes, increases one's social acceptance. Support groups run by self-help organizations frequently can be helpful initially with learning to cope with being different and not meeting the physical norms of society. Before one can take the first steps toward social recovery, however, she must make sure that her own attitudes about appearance, illness, and physical changes are not the same negative attitudes that many of her peers hold. If the person fails to recognize and fails to jettison her own prejudices about her worthiness, certainly she will have a much more difficult time in her attempts to rejoin her social circle. If she does not confront such prejudices, she may find herself staying away from the job or social events, which only increases the sense of isolation and aloneness.

This is what is happening to Madelyn in this vignette. She needs a family member or close friend to confront her tendency to stay at home and to help her return to work. She will need to make the first overtures to her colleagues at work. Possibly in the teacher's lounge, she can sit down with one or two of her fellow teachers and briefly discuss her problems, then move on to issues of mutual concern. They may be a great source of support. She needs to let them know what is wrong, but she does not need to dwell on her problem, and in this way she can quickly demonstrate that she is the same old Madelyn with the same old interests, etc. It is easier and more humanizing to do this reentering of one's social group by talking only to one or two people at a time, rather than arranging to speak, for example, to the whole teaching faculty at once. While this may reduce the number of times Madelyn has to talk about the disability, the advantage of one-to-one interaction in reassuring others that the illness has not destroyed the old Madelyn, is lost.

Students in her classes will be curious about her change in appearance and may harbor their own fears. She should acknowledge to them that she has experienced an illness, but that it is nothing for them to be concerned about and that she will continue as their teacher. She should give them the opportunity to ask questions if they have any concerns.

In addition, Madelyn might invite people who have avoided her, to have coffee with her to see if she can make them more comfortable if she takes the first step. Some people will respond, and others will be lost forever. However, some new friends might be made because of their ability to respond in a caring and helpful way at work, and these will likely be more lasting and dependable friends.

It is necessary to be aggressive about your rights to participate and be included in things. Physical disability is not a reason to be excluded from social conversations or from group social events. If people don't come up to you, go up to them. It is your responsibility to assertively remind people of your needs, so that they do not forget and you can participate with them. Then you will feel a part of things. For example, if you are wheelchair bound, and an after-work event is being planned, make sure the place that is picked is accessible. Do not sit back waiting to see if your coworkers remember that you need an accessible place. When you do that, it is a test that they might fail, but the real loser will be you, because you will be left out unnecessarily.

◆ Madelyn and Rob had planned to marry in about six months, when her paralysis occurred. Now she had great difficulty relating to Rob, as she felt ugly and did not want to burden him with her self-doubts. Sometimes she felt embarrassed for herself and for him. For example, eating out had been a favorite date for them, but now it was almost torture for her; she had to watch every bite she ate, because bits of food had a tendency to fall out of the paralyzed corner of her mouth. Sometimes Madelyn felt Rob was staying with her because he felt he had a duty to. Rob, on the other hand, was feeling shut out and unwanted; he loved Madelyn, but she did not seem to want to share her feelings with him.

Two people in a relationship are partners. They have to problem solve during the good times and bad times. The physical changes have become foremost in Madelyn's mind and have overshadowed the fact that in a caring, love relationship, more is shared than physical beauty and perfect, sanitized behavior. Neither Rob nor Madelyn should deny his or her feelings of frustration and despair, neither should they withdraw from the relationship because there is a physical problem. Rob and Madelyn need to try to develop a means of communication which would allow them to discuss what has happened and each of their feelings about it. One way they could do this, is for Rob to open up the conversation. It is sometimes easier for the nonafflicted spouse or boy/girlfriend to make the first move. One evening at Madelyn's or his home, he might say to her, "Madelyn, I would like to talk with you about your physical problem. I sometimes think you don't want to be with me anymore. You don't seem to want to do the things you liked doing before. Does it have to do with your illness? Or does it have to do with your feelings toward me? Tell me so that we can work it out." If a nonafflicted spouse or boy/girlfriend feels it is too upsetting to bring up these things, or if it is not their style to discuss emotional or disturbing things, then the ill person needs to do it. Madelyn could say, for example, "Rob, I have been feeling terrible lately. Have you noticed a difference in me? I feel very unattractive and think I might be a burden to you. If you want out of this relationship, let's talk about it. It would hurt me a lot, but I think I would rather have that, than have you pity me or hate me."

These conversation lead-ins usually work. Once they have started talking, even if the response of a loved one is the ill person's worst fantasy, there can be some resolution other then tense silences, angry outbursts, or nonunderstandable withdrawal. Once conversations have been opened up, then they can continue so that the couple can talk about other issues and priorities. For example, what activities can they continue to mutually participate in? If eating out is too difficult right now for Madelyn, then perhaps they can bring food home or take turns cooking at home and inviting some close friends over to enjoy the food with them.

Illness and disability do not prevent the sharing of one's intellect and displaying one's capacity to love. If Rob cannot accept the physical changes or the changes in life-style, then the relationship is better ended; there are many men to whom perfect physical beauty is a secondary consideration. The ending of a relationship under these conditions can be sad and painful, but is not an indication that one cannot love or be loved. It is very important to focus on what can be done and on one's abilities, rather than on what is lost or no longer a choice.

◆ After a few heart-to-heart discussions, Madelyn and Rob were able to get things together, and by working at it, re-established some of their former close relationships with other teachers who now seemed to accept her as she was. However, Madelyn was very hurt by the actions of Rob's mother who had treated her as a daughter for nearly the entire five years the two had dated. Not only had the relationship seemed to sour now that Madelyn's appearance had changed, Rob's mother seemed to avoid any mention of the paralysis or of the wedding. This made conversations very strained and few and far between. Since Madelyn's own mother had been dead for many years, she had treasured this relationship, and the loss of it was very painful.

Parents want everything to be perfect for their children. When things do not turn out that way, it can be very difficult for them not only to acknowledge the problem, but also to find positive ways to cope. The easiest way to cope is by avoiding the subject and pretending nothing had changed. There is concealed in this the futile hope that if it is ignored, the illness or injury will go away. The net result of this approach is always pain and frustration for all involved. The family experiencing the medical problem is doing its best to cope. If the near relatives refuse to acknowledge the illness, it is impossible for the suffering family to get the support and reassurance for which they are desperate. If an in-law or other relative (cousins, siblings, aunts and uncles, etc.) who has been close with the family prior to the illness, finds he is unable to face the problem and is abandoning the family, he needs to examine his own feelings and try to come to terms with the reason. If one's own family treats you as if you are an outcast, how can you expect the rest of the world to act differently? Inevitably, if this is the course the extended family takes, the relationship between the families will suffer.

Sometimes the problem is more complex than it seems on the surface. The family member who is ignoring the problem may have difficulty in talking about serious issues. Rob's mother, in our vignette, may not want to talk about the paralysis, because she is having so much trouble adjusting that she is afraid she will say something insensitive and hurt Madelyn's feelings. She may feel embarrassed about being seen with or related to someone with the paralysis and feel guilty about that embarrassment.

Rob's mother may have an irrational fear—that even she does not understand—that because her son is associating with an ill person, something similar may happen to him or that this now imperfect woman is no longer the correct mate for her son. She may also be afraid that there will be something wrong with future children, and thus may find herself secretly wishing that her son not marry Madelyn. Whatever the difficulty, it is important for Madelyn to talk with her future mother-in-law. Rob's mother will likely be unable to bring up the subject for fear of hurting Madelyn's feelings or because of the rush of unpleasant feelings she is afraid might occur in herself. If Madelyn can initiate the conversation, she, in effect, breaks the myth that by not talking about it or thinking about it, it will go away.

As in many situations, the burden of effort falls on the affected person. It will help Madelyn to be able to speak to Rob's mother, and speaking together may help to reestablish the relationship. If it is at all possible, Madelyn needs to try to talk with her future mother-in-law to try to reestablish their previously good relationship. However, if it looks like this is not going to be easy, perhaps Rob could talk to his mother first so she might be able to voice her fears and explain her withdrawal to him. Rob then can at least have a chance to reassure his mother or suggest outside help for her if it looks like this would help her cope better. If Rob is successful, then maybe Rob's mother and Madelyn will be able to talk about their sadness and sense of grief about the changes. It could be very helpful to both of them if they could talk about their fears about the future together, and if Madelyn could let Rob's mother know how much their relationship means to her and how much she would miss not having it. If Madelyn and Rob's mother can communicate, then Madelyn can have someone to talk to and someone who can be an additional support for her. Rob's mother might provide some physical help at home with cooking and household chores, or with shopping, as well as provide moral support at doctors' appointments like Madelyn's own mother might have done were she alive.

Madelyn may also have to see how this goes and face the possibility that Rob's mother may not be able to overcome her fears and prejudices. Then she and Rob have to talk and decide if they can deal with an estranged relationship with his mother. If Rob's mother is willing to cooperate, the three of them could go for brief counseling to try and resolve the conflict. However, if that doesn't work, then the relationship between Madelyn and Rob has to be strong enough to sustain the conflict. Hopefully in time, and with the coming of grandchildren, if that is what is decided, Rob's mother will be able to be part of the family again. It is important for Rob and Madelyn to always leave the door open for his mother.

Parents who find themselves in conflicts like this need to ask themselves if the uncompromising stand they have elected to take is worth the losses they will endure and the pain they will ultimately cause their children. Many times parents do not think far enough into the future to realize what might be at stake if they cannot resolve some of the distressing feelings that illness of this type creates. For Rob's mother, it could be the loss of a relationship with her son and future grandchildren. Perhaps counseling will not seem so terrible when the consequences are clearly stated.

Rob may have to say to his mother, "Mom, I don't want this to happen, but if you cannot come to grips with your feelings and accept Madelyn, then I am going to have to see you less often. I love Madelyn, and it makes me very unhappy to see the way you are treating her. If for no other reason than for me, please find a way to resolve this behavior. If you don't, then I will be forced to choose Madelyn over you. I will not give Madelyn up." Hopefully, this type of confrontation will help Rob's mother get help and resolve her feelings so that she can have some kind of relationship with her future daughter-in-law. Frequently, this kind of limit-setting of parents does work and is appropriate for the child to do. Madelyn does not need to do it. It is Rob's mother, and he has to establish the boundaries and set the limits. This setting of ground rules also supports Madelyn and enhances their relationship.

Leo

◆ Leo was confined to a wheelchair after his motorcycle rammed a bridge abutment. They said he was lucky to survive, but now a year later he was quite convinced he would have been luckier dead. A paraplegic, he has good use of his hands and has all the special equipment he needs to be independent. Despite this and the fact that he has a car with hand controls, he now spends nearly all day every day in his special first-floor apartment watching TV and eating. He had gained fifty pounds since the accident and rarely answered calls from his old friends or made any effort to see them. He could not do the kind of things they liked now anyway.

Difficulty accepting the changes that a serious disability brings on can result in apathy and withdrawal. It is this kind of withdrawal that can bring social isolation. Frequently in rehabilitation centers, associations like the Canadian Paraplegic Association, the Paralyzed Veterans Organizations, and the American Heart, or Diabetes Association make contact with patients and their families (social workers, doctors, psychologists, will know of such organizations). Through these associations, social contacts with other persons afflicted in the same way can begin. These associations offer many services. The American Heart Association offers many programs. Heart and stroke clubs are numerous and offer educational and social monthly meetings for persons who have suffered heart attacks or strokes, and their families. Caring-for-Your-Heart Programs are structured support programs for persons who have had a cardiac- or stroke-related problem and their families. Parents and Cardiac Children Together is another program offering education and support for parents of children with congenital or acquired heart defects offered through the American Heart Association. Paralyzed veterans organizations offer many services such as wheelchair repair service, sports and recreation, benefits service, social services, and planning and design for home renovations. It is by exposure to others with similar problems that one learns what is possible. Then with practice and experimentation, one can learn what one's individual potential is and try to reach it. These associations not only provide services but also allow this kind of socialization with peers. (See Appendix 1.)

For many people, the initial months or years after an injury or permanent stable disability like a stroke are times of adjusting and gaining confidence. As confidence grows, it becomes possible to explore options. As this happens, it reinforces confidence. By having goals and pursuing goals, one meets new friends, and new social groups develop. As with anyone—well or not—finding activities, jobs, and support groups takes some initiative and time. It does not just fall into your lap. No one is going to reward you for sitting around and feeling sorry for yourself, and no one is going to make the first moves for you.

Regardless of the cause of disability (amputation for diabetic vasculopathy, the result of a brain abscess or tumor, stroke paralysis, or cerebral palsy, to name a few), you must take the initiative; there is nothing to lose. Once you begin, usually it is surprising to learn how acceptable you are to many people and how much more you can do than you thought you could do. Travel is another possibility, and there are many travel agents who manage travel plans for the disabled. Many cities have listings of accessible museums, parks, and activities. *The Spinal Network,* by Sam Maddox, is a publication that lists activities for the disabled, such as aerobic exercises in the chair, sports, recreation, and travel. Networking with organizations that focus on the needs of the disabled, as well as gathering all the literature available, is one step toward moving out and back into the world.

◆ Leo contacted a chapter of the paralyzed veterans association since he was a veteran, and with their help, he was able to get a job in the parts department of a motorcycle dealership. Feeling much more sure of himself, Leo lost his extra weight and soon after met Cindy. He hopes that they will marry in the near future.

There is a future for persons with illness and disability, if everything can be put into perspective and one does not become consumed by the disability. If the ill or disabled person's problem becomes the center of his life, no one will want to be around him. It is important to learn balance. Life is fragile and difficult under the best of circumstances. Each of us has some cross to bear; while for some it might be much greater than for others, it is never all there is to life.

It is easy to idealize life prior to injury or illness and assume that everything was perfect then, and to believe that there were no worries about jobs, or finding spouses, or family arguments, or making friends. It becomes a mythical time when we pretend that everything was perfect. The fact is that most people had basically the same personalities before their illness or injury as after, and probably had the same problems then, though one's particular personality traits (e.g., shyness) may now make some tasks more difficult.

No matter what the physical condition of any of us, we have to make an effort to reach our goals. The first step is to decide what it is you want to do. What is most important to know is that in doing this, there are many choices available to each of us, regardless of what the problem is. But it does take some effort to sit down and search out the best way to reach goals, to call organizations or people who might be of help, and to follow through with their suggestions. A family member or friend might be asked to help you initially make contact. Don't be embarrassed to ask for this kind of help. Have a family member or friend go with you to the appropriate association. Find out what interests you and what other people are doing. Ask questions of people who are there and who are running the groups or services. Tell them what you need and what you see as your problems. These people have information and ideas, and sometimes can offer you a job or suggest a volunteer activity. Try out sports and recreation if that was one of the things you loved to do. The list of available sports for the disabled is impressively long. Try out many different things before you make up your mind. It might take some trial and error before you find the things that make you want to get up in the morning. Give yourself time to find the right activities. Organizations and groups that can help you are listed in Appendix 1.

The disabled person, like anyone, can have the kind of life that brings love and a sense of purpose to each day. It will not be a life that is trouble free and without disappointments. Not even the able-bodied have that! The most important thing is for the person to acknowledge his own self-worth by looking for activities and social possibilities, and then to recognize opportunities to reach goals and to take advantage of opportunities when they are there.

Raymond

◆ Raymond at thirty-eight had worked his way up to a middle management position in an insurance firm after fourteen years of working as a commissioned salesman. His pride in this accomplishment, however, was tempered by the recent discovery in his longtime partner, John, of HIV infection. Raymond was in his new position for only a few months when the unthinkable happened. He began to notice a reddish, purple rash on his arms and trunk. The doctor confirmed his worst fears. It was a form of cancer, Kaposi's Sarcoma, that is common in AIDS; Raymond had AIDS. The news spread quickly. Despite his trying to hide the spots with long-sleeved shirts, Raymond's coworkers seemed to all know his diagnosis. He was not asked to coffee or lunch much any more. One day his immediate boss suggested he quit and go on disability. Raymond was taken aback. Though he had AIDS, he still felt well and knew he was doing a good job. He was beginning to feel pushed out and ostracized by his previously friendly colleagues.

A primary and pervasive force underlying the insidious social isolation of persons suffering from HIV infection and AIDS is the fears of co-workers, friends, and family, that association with the person will result in contamination. This fear and the resulting ostracism continue, despite the extensive research and educational efforts that have been made to educate the public to the fact that the AIDS virus is *not* spread through normal social contact at work, in the community, or at home, or through using toilets or sinks that a person infected with the AIDS virus has used. Many people are so terrified of becoming infected with this virus that they consider to be a virtual death sentence, that they believe any contact or even being near someone with the infection is risky. These beliefs and the emotions accompanying them, are often so strongly held that any amount of research or documentation is unlikely to change the behavior of the person holding the beliefs.

Simply being publicly identified as a homosexual or an IV drug user is sometimes a stigma in a particular work or social situation. Being labeled as such may sometimes result in loss of friends, business contacts, or even loss of jobs. If coworkers, employers, and friends first find out about one's private life when the ravages of the AIDS virus are apparent, the person may be subjected to even more rejection, anger, and embarrassment.

Many people also find it very difficult to deal with the realization that someone near their own age and with whom they work and are friends, is going to die. Seeing this person on a daily basis makes coworkers face their own mortality and causes anxiety about the anticipated loss of that person and the pain of living through his death. It is much easier for coworkers to handle this pain by distancing themselves from the ill person by excluding him from daily social contact.

Raymond's boss is most likely to be fearful about the effects on Raymond's work and attendance. Employers may be concerned about infection, but they also worry about the demoralizing effects on other employees, the loss of time and energy which would result in lowered productivity, and the effects of all of this on their business or their own productivity in the company. However, as indicated in this vignette, it is premature to ask Raymond to leave. With proper medical management, he can work productively for a long time. Working will be psychologically very important for him. It will allow him to maintain some social network and to feel productive in spite of his devastating diagnosis.

Here are some things that Raymond can do to make his life more satisfying and enjoyable:

1. Get support from Gay Men's Health Organizations. Attend support groups and talk about what is happening at work. This diagnosis may be a death sentence, so there are feelings of fear, sadness, and anger, which must accompany it. Not everyone needs to talk about these feelings, but seeking help to cope with the diagnosis and the consequences on one's work and relationships, is a first step. It is important to talk about the stigma of the disease and share ways to avoid social isolation.

2. Get a physician who is familiar with treating AIDS patients and has access to current information about medical management. Participate in studies, if possible (see Chapter 7: Coping with Depression), which are testing new medications or treatments. Stay on top of the latest information.

3. Talk with your boss. Try to educate him to the facts and let him know that it is important to you to be able to remain working as long as possible. Sometimes bosses think they are doing you a favor if they give you early disability, though this is rarely a good idea. If your work suffers, then discussions about retirement can begin. Various alternatives for part-time work may be possible, or for alternative responsibilities on the job, and these alternatives can be discussed with your boss. (See Chapter 14: Handling Changes at Work.)

4. Discuss with friends, family, and lovers what the options financially are. Can you go on partial disability? Is insurance covering medications and hospitalizations? These costs can be prohibitively expensive. Try to locate physicians and pharmacies that are charging lower or discounted prices. Contact the National AIDS Network Agency or the National AIDS Hot Line to get all the information about medications and where to get them, availability of support services, legal information, and treatment information.

5. Locate service programs funded by state health departments which include crisis intervention, social work services, and counseling. Many of these programs also offer legal services, a buddy program, and hospital visits. Contact your state health department and the Red Cross to find out what services are available to you.

◆ John and Raymond were both outgoing and had enjoyed a full social life. Both had also kept close contact with their respective families. Raymond's family, who had always had difficulty accepting his homosexuality, now seemed to be shutting him out. While his parents and sister still called at least once a week, they rarely dropped by the apartment anymore. He found out about a cousin's wedding only by accident and did not receive an invitation. Being dropped by his family hurt almost as much as the disease.

John's family, on the other hand, was at first both shocked and devastated by his infection and Raymond's disease. However, once they were able to grasp the situation, they were very supportive to both men. Not only did John's parents continue to include the men in their social activities, but John's mother also became active in an organization of relatives of people with HIV infection and AIDS.

It is deeply sad when family support disappears because of prejudice, shame, or embarrassment. Families that cannot accept their children's homosexuality often experience it as a negative reflection on them (sometimes family members, usually mothers, feel they caused the homosexuality) and a deep embarrassment. Fathers may feel deep shame and anger that their son is "not a man." Sometimes the feelings are driven by religious beliefs that homosexuality is wrong in the eyes of God and to be homosexual is to commit an unforgivable sin. Families that feel this way have usually kept their child's homosexuality a secret or tried to deny the truth by never talking about it in the vain hope that if it were not talked about, it might go away. In these families, the diagnosis of AIDS causes tremendous difficulty. Not only is there the pain of possibly losing a child, but there is the sense that *everyone* will now know, and the profound embarrassment this realization causes. It can often feel like the child—or indeed the family—is being punished because of the homosexuality.

Family support is an important factor in the course of any illness, whether it is AIDS or asthma! People with strong family support often recover faster from operations and illnesses. Raymond's burdens could be greatly lessened if he had the support of his family and could share his pain with them. Just knowing they could put aside their prejudices and were behind him would help him get through the ups and downs of his unpredictable disease.

If he cannot educate his family through literature or through talking to them, perhaps he can suggest they go into counseling together. Raymond may also need to rely more on John's family. He may be able to ask John's parents to have his parents over to talk to them. Maybe they can go with John's parents to one of the meetings for relatives that John's parents attend.

If Raymond's family can overcome their shame and guilt, they could be of great help to him through the next very difficult years. It would be an opportunity for all of them to resolve many of the unfinished conflicts from the past, and when his death did come, he and his family could feel at peace with each other.

Stephanie

◆ Stephanie, the honor student. Stephanie, the gymnast. Stephanie, the cheerleader. Stephanie was a popular, outgoing fifteen-year-old. But when she developed Hodgkins Disease, a form of lymph-node cancer, her young world turned upside down. She had to undergo a series of radiation treatments and chemotherapy. These made her feel very fatigued and sometimes quite ill. Some of her hair fell out, and she lost weight. She felt ugly, and for several months, she could not go to school.

After about a year, the doctors told her that all signs of the cancer were gone and they were hopeful of a full recovery. Her hair was growing back and looked shiny and healthy, and she was regaining some weight. However, Stephanie had become a virtual homebody. Her parents did all they could for her, even to the point of neglecting the needs of her two younger sisters at times, and encouraged her to stay home and take care of herself in hopes that the cancer would not come back. Stephanie wanted to go out more but was embarrassed about being different, and she worried that the other kids would avoid her and talk about her.

Soon most of her friends were off doing other things, and Stephanie saw little of them. They no longer came by to see her, and she made no effort to get out of the house to see them. Since she was now sixteen, she decided to drop out of school and just stay at home. It seemed a lot easier than trying to get back in with the crowd she used to hang around with, and she felt secure at home. Maybe later on, she would take some correspondence courses and finish high school.

Because of her illness, Stephanie had to stop the world and step off. Now that she is in remission and can think about her future, it seems as if she does not know how to or is afraid to get back on. The maturation process for her has been disturbed. Teenagers begin the long and difficult process of separation from their parents and home during these adolescent years. Because of her illness and because her parents wanted to protect her, Stephanie has stopped separating and developing her own individual life. She needs to begin that process again. Now is the time for her parents to support her. She needs them *not* to collude with her plans not to continue in school, but rather to step in and stop her from dropping out of school. Not only should they insist that she stay in school, but they should also insist that she plan to go away to college as she would have if she had not developed the disease. If they believe she can handle it emotionally, she will believe it; if they encourage her and work with her to reenter her social world, she will be able to.

It is very frightening and overwhelming for parents to have a child develop a life-threatening disease. Not only is it painful, but it seems to go against the natural order of things. Parents are supposed to become ill and die first.

When a child survives a life-threatening situation, parents who have felt the indescribable pain of nearly losing that child can become over-cautious and try in the best ways they know how to protect and shield him. Unfortunately, these well-intentioned efforts are often not in the adolescent's best interests, because they tend to keep him in a child role and prevent him from growing up. It is very important for parents to fight these strong impulses to protect, because an adolescent needs the support of his family to handle the difficult social situations that this age brings, even when there is no illness to complicate things. If the child knows he will be treated like a child rather than recognized as a maturing adolescent, he may not feel comfortable with his parents and will not be able to call upon them for the support he needs.

It is very hard to be different in any way at this age; that's why all teenagers dress alike and talk alike. Even without the added factor of illness, teenagers suffer fears of rejection. With the stigma of a serious illness that has slowed down activities and studies, the teenager may well resort to refuge in his secure home, and his outlook for normal development is particularly precarious.

Now is the time for Stephanie's parents to call the school and speak with the guidance counselors and teachers so that everyone will encourage Stephanie to participate. The school can be very helpful at this time. It might be a good idea for Stephanie to join an adolescent group in the community to share her fears and see how other teenagers are responding to her. She might also do some volunteer work in the community just to begin building her confidence. She might even consider going to work after school. Local chapters of the Cancer Society often have support groups of young patients who have fought cancer and are now trying to live normal lives.

It is very important to begin living as normal a life as possible when illness or disability has stabilized. If Stephanie's parents are having too difficult a time, they might benefit from joining groups run by the Cancer Society for parents who have children with a diagnosis of cancer. These support groups may help them see what their role needs to be at this time. Also, talking with a counselor may help them learn how to help Stephanie get back on track.

◆ There are people who are willing to be a part of one's life, and there are activities that are appropriate for participation by ill and disabled persons. Being active and being with other people is the most important way to avoid feelings of despair and loneliness.

◆ Close friends should be taken into your confidence and told about the illness or disabilities so that they can help.

◆ Talk about your feelings and the fears associated with loss of self-esteem and prestige.

◆ Most people simply do not know what to say or how to act around someone who is ill or disabled. The job of making them feel comfortable falls to the ill or disabled person and his/her family.

- Join local church-run groups or church-run activities, attend illness-related support groups to learn more, interact with people with similar problems, and meet new people.

- If traveling was a part of one's life before illness or disability, it can be part of one's life again. Look at *Frommer's Guide for the Disabled Traveler.* (Appendix 2)

- It is necessary to be aggressive about your rights to participate and be included in things. It is your responsibility to remind people of your needs so they do not forget, and you can participate with them.

- When the ill or disabled person and his/her family talk about their own feelings about illness and disability and start to recognize and overcome negative attitudes about disability and illness that they all have, it makes it easier to form friends and socialize.

- When an ill or disabled partner or friend is withdrawing and not talking about what is wrong, the well partner, relative, or friend may need to open the conversation and make the first move. Don't be afraid of embarrassing or hurting the ill or disabled person's feelings. You are doing them a favor in the long run.

- It is easy to idealize life before illness or disability and to assume that everything was perfect then and to believe that there were no worries about jobs, or finding spouses, or family arguments, or making friends. The truth is that there were problems then too. Now the important thing is to recognize that there are many choices available, recognize opportunities to reach goals, and take advantage of them.

CHAPTER 17

Building a New Dream

"Life with a disability (or illness) doesn't have to be any way, except the way that you make it. Sure, there are in reality things that one can't do anymore, but if you can't do it that way, there's another way you can approximate doing most anything you want to. If you keep trying, if you are active, if you keep yourself exposed to other people, if you seek stimulation of one sort or the other, you're gonna get rewarded for it."
George Hohmann (*Options: Spinal Cord Injury and the Future*, Barry Corbet)

Our plans and dreams for the future are often turned upside down when illness or disability intercedes. Career ambitions may be thwarted; at worst, illness or injury may cause total disability. Dreams of accomplishment, financial gain, watching one's children grow up, playing sports with them, or of traveling around the world following an early retirement are suddenly shattered.

And as if the loss of the future were not enough, the person may find himself physically disabled with some pain, and the family and spouse may be faced with the unanticipated burden of his care. Facing this prospect, anyone in the family might well feel resentment, anger, and frustration.

Every family has a dream of the future. Since every family member shares in this dream, and the loss is suffered by all family members, it can be the most profound loss of all. The second most profound insult comes from society: it is the often insensitive reaction of the well and able-bodied world. Picking up the pieces and starting to build a new dream is a crucial step in coping with and adapting to illness. It is "learning to live with it." Those who are able to do this can lead happy and fulfilling lives, despite their limitations.

Accommodations can be made so that a sick person and his family can continue most social activities. When physical disability, fatigue, or emotional factors make major changes necessary, new, appropriate activities that are fulfilling, yet take into account the disability, will need to be developed. For example, a previously avid tennis player with arthritis may be able with the aid of assistants, to become a tennis coach at a local recreational facility. Options may need to be pointed out to the ill person who may have difficulty recognizing alternatives in the face of pain and the mourning of his/her losses. One may be forced to construct alternative ways of participation in family interactions and work relationships as well.

The point of this chapter is to focus the energies of the individual and family toward developing new goals as this can and must be done for the family unit to be maintained and continue to have a fulfilling life together. Foregoing old and now unattainable plans for a more meaningful future can help to maintain the family cohesiveness and enrich the lives of all members. It is our belief that the ill or disabled person can maintain an active and satisfying life and can redesign the future to build new dreams in the image of the old dreams. In this chapter, we will give some suggestions as to how plans can be modified to incorporate some of the lost dreams.

To feel capable of and motivated to redesign the future, to reformulate personal and family goals, and to maintain an active life, frequent family discussions with all the involved people are necessary. You must decide you want to do this and are going to do it with their help and with their suggestions.

◆ One morning after they had had breakfast, Jan went to Mel and told him she wanted to speak to him alone. Taking a deep breath, Jan began, "Mel, I know we have lost a lot in the way of our future hopes and plans. I would like to work with you to plan how we want our life to be now. I need your help. I cannot work all day and take care of all the housework and errands when I get home. It would be a great help to me if you could work with the house-keeper. For instance, a real time-saver would be if you could go shopping for the groceries or make up a menu for the week that the housekeeper can use to go shopping. Could you take our six-year-old to his after-school activities? Also, I want to talk to you about the future. I want us to enjoy life despite what has happened. I want a plan for our daily life and a plan for our social life. Let's talk about what we can still do together and with whom we can still socialize."

This may sound hard to do, but it helps to know that, in reality, in most families each person is waiting for the other to do or say something. The hardest conversations to initiate seem to be those about planning and actively redesigning the way family members live their lives together. The most common reason each person will have for not speaking first is the misconception that they will hurt or embarrass the other.

The hardest part may be actually getting the discussions started, but that is still only the beginning; there is still a lot of work to do. You have to look at changes caused by the illness and decide what plans are irreparable, what can remain in place with modifications, and what can continue unaltered. Then you must decide and agree upon what the changes will be. It is important to focus on present abilities and not on what can no longer be done—the disabilities.

It may not be easy; life probably wasn't easy before. You may feel scared or anxious, but many able-bodied and well people feel anxious when considering their futures. We all have the capacity to feel several emotions at once; it is possible to feel scared and anxious and to still push forward with your life. It is not fair to you or your family to accept less for yourself because you are sick or disabled, if you could do otherwise. If you do not want to do certain things because you are not interested in them, it is possible to choose something else, as you might have done before you became ill or disabled. You may have to search out new ways to do old things, but keep doing the things you enjoy as long as you possibly can. Ask yourself, "If I liked it before, did it before, and can still do it now, then why aren't I doing it now?"

A lawyer with deforming arthritis can no longer go to the office, but can practice from his home with a computer and devices that will allow him to use the computer. He can hire a partner or his spouse, or use his children. He can advertise for teenagers interested in a law career, or employ relatives who have free time and who can run around to the libraries and to the courthouse. Together they can work on the ideas and plan the strategies. The substance of his work is now more intellectual and planning than physical, but it gets done. This can be true regardless of the nature of the illness or its disabling aspects. Look at your skills; what can you still do? If you need legs, hands, a secretary, or someone to climb stairs, hire them. Turn to family and neighbors.

Many people who are retired, work part-time or not at all, would love some small daily task to do. Blind people use readers to help them, and it works very well. In fact, a reader job is the kind of job someone can do if he/she no longer can work as the result of an injury or disabling illness and wants to feel useful.

Maximize your strengths. If you are a carpenter, painter, or handyman, who after a heart attack can no longer work the long hours or lift the heavy materials necessary in construction work, then think about smaller jobs in the neighborhood. You can advertise in local, neighborhood papers. You can also train or supervise. Your knowledge is in your head and in your mind's eye; your hands may be replaced, but your creativity and knowledge cannot be. You can share your knowledge either by training or teaching. You can find a job which would allow you to do this for money, or you can volunteer. Do not spend time focusing on what is no longer possible. Use that energy to focus on what you can still do. You are limited only by your own unwillingness or failure to take advantage of opportunities.

Sit down with a spouse or a friend, someone with good ideas who can help you focus on what you can do. Take a pencil and paper and make a list. Use your imagination. It is amazing the things people take for granted that they do which are marketable skills and alternative activities still available to them. Think about hobbies and activities you did when you were on vacation or on the weekends.

For example, you might play the guitar and have played it for years. All of a sudden, as the result of a severe heart attack, you can no longer work or enjoy your usual games of tennis. However, you can give guitar lessons. You can record your own songs and teach others how to write music. What once was a hobby can now be a job.

◆ Joe was an architect when he got the news that he had Parkinson's Disease. At first the tremors were controlled with medication. Eventually, he could not hold a pencil steady enough to do the blueprints. He investigated and bought a computer with a program for architects. For a while he could do his blueprints with the computer. Soon it became very difficult for him to work at all, and he had to retire. At home he felt lost and useless. His brother-in-law, however, had just bought some property. He wanted help designing a home and asked Joe to help. This project allowed Joe to be active. He designed in his head and used a draftsman to have it put on paper. After that, Joe spoke to the town board and was invited to sit on the architectural planning committee. He also volunteered to help other family members and friends design bathrooms or porches on their homes.

Joe is adapting and actively using his skills. He is beginning to redesign his future in a way that is fulfilling to him. He is actively thinking of new ways that he can have an active life. In addition to the ideas in the vignette, Joe might have been able to teach or buy property for himself and design something for his family. He might also redesign things in his own home, like the bathroom or kitchen.

Think about your previous hopes and plans. If travel was in your future, then look at the ways you can still travel. You may no longer be able to go to underdeveloped, unpopulated islands with little in the way of hospital and medical facilities, but you certainly can travel to other places. Make a list of the new places to which you would like to go. Look up the accessibility of hotels, restaurants, and beaches, and talk with physicians about medical facilities which are available. If you have to give up some plans, pick the next best thing that is still available.

If you liked skiing or boating, but because of amputations can no longer ski, investigate other sports or alternate ways to ski. There are special devices which can make skiing a viable option. Boating for the disabled is also an option. Check with local associations about wheelchair sports. (See Appendix 1.)

You may have to give up some spontaneity. Jumping in the car and taking off without a plan or a care may no longer be possible, but this is a small price to pay. In the face of disability, planning ahead becomes an important component of being able to maintain a satisfying life. If you have a diagnosis of any illness which may progressively debilitate you, sit down with the family and plan for future needs. Do you want to have a child? Do you want to move to a home without stairs in a warmer climate? Do you want to go back to school now or get retrained? Do you need to think about insurance for nursing needs, medication, and supplies? If you are a veteran, have you joined veterans' associations that will help you prepare for future needs? If the worst happened and there were hospitalizations, supplies, and medication costs, how would you pay for them and still have money to educate your children or retire?

Speak to health-care professionals to learn all about your current and future limitations, and lawyers to learn about the possible financial and legal complications and options. Talk to all family members including brothers, sisters, parents, in-laws, cousins, aunts, uncles, etc. How can any of them help? How can they be included in the future plans?

Plan for current and future caretakers to have activities of their own so that they will not become emotionally exhausted, but also include activities that the ill or disabled person can participate in to avoid social isolation for the whole family. Even though with many disabling illnesses, there are personality changes that make the person fearful, depressed, and angry, progress can be made toward a useful and satisfying life. It is easier when illness stabilizes, or when disabling treatments are finished, to plan the future. However, it is important to consider future plans and modifications even during acute phases of illness or during treatments that are unpleasant. Thinking about the future brings a sense of control and the promise of better days.

Sometimes it is hard to maintain the motivation and positive attitudes that are necessary to complete the strenuous job of redesigning one's life. Here are a few important points to remember so you will not become discouraged and can overcome negative forces, feel energized, and press onward toward your goals.

1. The able-bodied and well world is very intolerant and frightened by illness and disability. Expectations are lowered for the ill and disabled, and discrimination does occur. It is easy for you to be placed in an invalid role and treated as an invalid even though you are not. It is the disabled and ill person's job not to permit others to infantilize them. Throughout this book, we have emphasized the importance of being active, maintaining high expectations for oneself, and avoiding the unnecessary and demoralizing role of an invalid. Maintaining a sense of self and dignity requires that others not be allowed to do things for the ill person that he can do for himself or herself. It is very important not to treat ill children as if they are so different from well children, and most of all they should not be allowed to dictate the family's future. Siblings must be able to live their lives guilt-free. It is the parents' responsibility not to reinforce guilt feelings on well siblings who are not responsible for the illness. Expectations, though possibly altered from before, must be maintained for the ill child who should not be allowed to become an invalid.

Despite society's obstacles, like poor wheelchair access, patronization, and at times cruelty, it is possible to utilize your potential and capability to the maximum to do most anything you choose to do. It is very painful to be devalued by society, and it requires even greater self-esteem and independence than when one is well, to ignore the devaluation. The able-bodied and healthy world does not want to feel vulnerable and to think about the fragility of life. That world would like all people who are injured or ill to keep their feelings about their losses to themselves and never complain. The imperfect are not supposed to upset anyone. Persons with illnesses, disabling illnesses, or injuries, know that they must not show their feelings of fear, sorrow, sexuality, or anger, for this disturbs and creates anxiety for the non-ill and able-bodied. This means that the ill and disabled must put on a "stiff upper lip." Although there are individual and cultural differences in regard to expressing feelings and talking about sadness and anger, when society takes away the choice, this, in and of itself, is infuriating. But practically speaking, you are unlikely to influence attitudes of society toward the ill and disabled as a group. What you can do is find friends and family members who see you as an individual and with whom you are able to share your feelings. You can find ways to express your rage. It is our hope that if you want to express your feelings, that reading this will give you permission to do so.

2. Some friends and some family members will not come around anymore. These are people who will not be able to handle the illness, the changes, and the feelings that accompany it. However, many other friends and family members will be able to remain friends. It is important for the spouse, and the ill or disabled person to speak to those friends and to nurture the relationships that exist. Loss of friends can be as much the fault of the suffering family as the friends. Invite them over to your house. If you do not continue to socialize, friends and family may not feel that they are still important; they may feel shut out. You should make the first move, as often friends feel they may be intruding or will hurt your feelings if they talk about you, your illness, or the things they love to do that you no longer can do. It is the ill or disabled person's job to make friends and family members comfortable with them and their illness. Explain to friends exactly what they are supposed to do to handle you physically, if they are willing to provide some care.

3. You will feel anger and sometimes rage after an illness, or injury, or accident. These feelings will come and go. They are expected. You certainly did not ask for this to happen, and it feels unfair and a terrible handicap. You may feel unlucky. You may feel frustration, sadness, and anger at life in general, and more specifically in those situations in which you can no longer do what was once possible. You may be jealous of those who are unafflicted, and you may be feeling affronted by the well and able-bodied world. You may have periods of trying to understand why this has happened. During these times, it is not unusual to think that it is a punishment for some misdeed or to feel responsible.

Take care that you do not become consumed by excessive blame or guilt which may impair your ability to function and live life. Assaults on one's self are painful, and the new, necessary self-identity may not be a welcome one. But that new person is a person who, while recognizing his limitations, can feel happiness, satisfaction, and pleasure. No one in life is guaranteed, whether able-bodied and healthy or not, that he will feel happy, satisfied, and have pleasure. There is a tendency to idealize the past, and oneself, and one's family in the past. It is not true that life was always wonderful. There were problems, pains, disappointments, and failures before injury or illness. There is no way of knowing how life would have been if injury or illness had not occurred.

4. Grieving may be mistaken for depression. Grieving is a normal, expected process when major, sad life events have occurred. Allow yourself, children, and family to grieve. If you can grieve together, all the better. Talking helps. Family members as well as the ill or disabled will also at times experience fears of dying. It is important to talk about these fears with clergy or family members and not to be embarrassed or afraid to do so. Sometimes fears about death lead to further planning for the future. Living wills might be important to consider, especially if one is concerned about experiencing pain or does not want to live on with life supports. This is the time to talk to family members about your wishes and to hear their opinions. It is also a way to decide whether or not there are some things you really want to do that have been left undone. Drawing up wills is so frequently left undone, because it causes so much anxiety for the family. Now may be a good time to think about your will. Also, there may be some unfinished business with family members, sisters, parents, children, or a spouse that, when thinking and talking about death, reminds one that he/she would like to do something about it. Children need an opportunity to talk with an ill or disabled parent so that their fears about their parent's death can be expressed. Children should not be protected from the facts, and from the expression of feelings. They do not need to be frightened unnecessarily, but they certainly know when something is going on, and they will respond better if they are allowed to express their feelings and opinions also. Frequently, diagnoses of AIDS or a recurrence of cancer brings a greater urgency to planning wills and a sense of immediacy and appropriateness to thoughts about death. However, even if the illness does not portend an imminent death, our associations of illness with impending death cause all members of the family to think about death. Surviving a massive heart attack, a serious accident, a mastectomy, brings a family and all its members closer to death than ever before. Talking about death and the consequences for the family allows families to make decisions and plans that they might never have had the opportunity to do otherwise. Speak with a lawyer or an estate planner. There may be things to do for the family that had never occurred to anyone before the illness struck. If grief or thoughts of death become disabling and debilitating to family members or the ill, then outside help may be needed to get to a place where functioning returns.

5. Sexuality can be part of your life. Sexuality is more than sexual intercourse. Sexuality is the expression of affection, warmth, and love. It is always possible to be sexual. It is always possible to give pleasure and feel pleasure. There are many ways to have an orgasm, and many ways to feel sexual pleasure. All of them are good. There is no one right way for anything. The choice is yours, and the decisions are yours. If you choose to have no sex in your life, then let it be a decision you make knowing that you have a choice. Being able to love and be loved, despite disabling illness or disability, allows persons afflicted with illnesses and disabilities to feel normal and human. Each of us in this world worries about our acceptability to others and our attractiveness. We worry about rejection and closeness, and meeting society's standards of beauty. The enormity of the cosmetic industry is evidence of this. For some reason, we forget this and tend to think that the disabled and ill are the only ones who are concerned with their differentness and acceptability. We make it their problem and suggest to them that they are no longer attractive enough to be loved and made love to. This is to deprive the ill or disabled of their right to feel normal. The ill or disabled do not have to accept this.

6. You can do whatever you want to do. This is the most important point to remember! You may have to alter the way you do it to fit the current abilities you have and to match the current restrictions on you, but with imagination, and family/friends' support, you can do it. Good luck!

◆ Maximize your strengths—focus on what you can still do.

◆ Be active, maintain high expectations for oneself, and avoid the unnecessary and demoralizing roles of an invalid.

◆ Many friends and family members will be able to be supportive and continue their relationships.

◆ You will feel anger and sadness after an illness, injury, or accident. These feelings will come and go.

◆ Grieving is a natural response to the losses brought on by the illness or disability.

◆ Sexuality can be a part of your life.

◆ You can do or be whatever you want to do or be.

Appendixes

Appendix 1

Listed below are centers, organizations, and associations that deal with many of the illnesses and disabilities referred to in the various vignettes throughout the book. Many other organizations dealing with other illnesses and disabilities are also included, as well as professional associations that can serve as a resource to the reader to help in selecting health professionals.

Associations also are often listed in the white pages of the telephone book under the name of the disease or organ involved. A very helpful publication located in the reference section of the library is the *Encyclopedia of Associations,* Michigan: Gale Research Inc., 23rd ed., 1989, Koek K., Martin S. B., and Novallo A., eds. This reference gives phone numbers, addresses, and descriptions of associations which include publications, convention meetings, councils, state, and local groups.

Gay Men's Health Crisis (AIDS)
Box 274
132 W. 24th St.
New York, NY 10011
(212) 807-7035

AIDS Committee of Toronto
66 Wellesley East
Toronto, Ontario
(416) 926-1626

National Association of People
  with AIDS
2025 I St. NW, Suite 415
Washington, DC 20006
(202) 429-2856

National AIDS Network
1012 14th St. NW, Suite 601
Washington, DC 20005
(202) 347-0390

Alzheimer's Disease and Related
  Disorders Association, Inc.
70 E. Lake St., Suite 600
Chicago, IL 60601
(312) 853-3060

Alzheimer Society of Canada
1320 Yonge St.
Suite 302
Toronto, Ontario, M4T1X2
(416) 925-3552

American Association of Retired
Persons
1909 K St. NW
Washington, DC 20049
(202) 872-4700

Canadian Association of Retired
Persons
27 Queen Street East
Toronto, Ontario
(416) 363-8748

American Cancer Society, Inc.
261 Madison Ave.
New York, NY 10016
(212) 599-3600

National Cancer Institute of
Canada
77 Bloor Street West
Toronto, Ontario
(416) 961-7223

American Diabetes Association
National Service Center
PO Box 25757
1660 Duke Street
Alexandria, VA 22313
(703) 549-1500

Canadian Diabetes Association
78 Bond Street
Toronto, Ontario
(416) 362-4440

American Foundation for the
Blind
15 W. 16th St.
New York, NY 10011
(212) 620-2000

Canadian Nat'l Institute for the
Blind
1931 Bayview Avenue
Toronto, Ontario
(416) 480-7580

American Heart Association
7320 Greenville Ave.
Dallas, TX 75231
(214) 373-6300

Canadian Heart Foundation
1 Nicholas Street, Suite 1200
Ottawa, Ontario
(613) 237-4361

American Liver Foundation
998 Pompton Ave.
Cedar Grove, NJ 07009
(201) 857-2626

Canadian Liver Foundation
42 Charles Street
Toronto, Ontario
(416) 964-1953

American Lung Association
(Respiratory Diseases)
1740 Broadway
New York, NY 10019
(212) 315-8700

Canadian Lung Association
75 Albert Street, Suite 908
Ottawa, Ontario
(613) 237-1208

American Nurses Association
2420 Pershing Rd.
Kansas City, MO 64108
(816) 474-5720

American Occupational Therapy
  Association
1383 Piccard Dr., Suite 301
Rockville, MD 20850
(301) 948-9626

American Parkinson's Disease
  Association
116 John St., Suite 417
New York, NY 10038
(212) 732-9550

Parkinson Foundation of Canada
55 Bloor Street West
Toronto, Ontario
(416) 964-1155

American Physical Therapy
  Association
1111 N. Fairfax St.
Alexandria, VA 22314
(703) 684-2782

American Psychiatric Association
1400 K St., NW
Washington, DC 20005
(202) 682-6000

American Psychological
  Association
1200 17th St., NW
Washington, DC 20036
(202) 955-7600

American Red Cross
17th and D Sts., NW
Washington, DC 20006
(202) 737-8300

Canadian Red Cross Society
95 Wellesley Street E.
Toronto, Ontario
(416) 923-6692

American Spinal Injury
  Association (Physicians)
250 E. Superior, Rm. 619
Chicago, IL 60611
(312) 908-3425

Spinal Cord Society of Canada
RR1
King City, Ontario
(416) 833-0984

Amyotrophic Lateral Sclerosis
  Association
15300 Ventura Blvd., Suite 315
Sherman Oaks, CA 91403
(818) 990-2151

Amyotrophic Lateral Sclerosis
  Society of Canada
250 Rogers
Toronto, Ontario
(416) 656-5242

Arthritis Foundation (Rheumatic
  Diseases)
1314 Spring St. NW
Atlanta, GA 30309
(404) 872-7100

Arthritis Society
250 Bloor Street E., #420
Toronto, Ontario
(416) 967-1414

Biomedical Engineering Centers:

Tufts-New England Medical
  Center
P.O. Box 1014
171 Harrison Ave.
Boston, MA 02111
(617) 956-5000

Texas Institute for Rehabilitation
  and Research
1333 Moursund Ave.
Houston, TX 77025
(713) 799-5000

Courage Center
3915 Golden Valley Rd.
Golden Valley, MN 55422
(612) 588-0811

University of Washington
School of Medicine
Department of Rehabilitation
  RJ-30
Seattle, WA 98195
(206) 543-1060

Cancer Care
1180 Avenue of the Americas
New York, NY 10036
(212) 221-3300

Cystic Fibrosis Foundation
6931 Arlington Rd., #200
Bethesda, MD 20814
(301) 951-4422

Cystic Fibrosis Foundation
586 Eglinton East
Toronto, Ontario
(416) 485-9149

Eastern Paralyzed Veterans
  Association
75-20 Astoria Blvd.
Queens, NY 11370-1178
(718) 803-3782

Canadian Paraplegic Association
520 Sutherland Drive
Toronto, Ontario
(416) 422-5640

Epilepsy Foundation of America
4351 Garden City Dr.
Landover, MD 20785
(301) 459-3700

Epilepsy Ontario
5385 Yonge Street
North York, Ontario
(416) 229-2291

Guillain-Barré Syndrome Support
   Group
P.O. Box 262
Wynnewood, PA 19096
(215) 649-7837

Heartlife (Cardiology)
P.O. Box 54305
Atlanta, GA 30308
(404) 523-0826

Huntington's Disease Society of
   America (Neurological
   disorders)
140 W 22nd St., 6th fr.
New York, NY 10011
(212) 242-1968

Huntington's Disease Resource
   Center
2175 Keele
North York, Ontario
(416) 656-8018

Leukemia Society of America,
   Inc.
733 Third Ave.
New York, NY 10017
(212) 573-8484

Lupus Foundation of America
11921 Olive Blvd.
St. Louis, MO
(314) 872-9036

Ontario Lupus Association
250 Bloor Street E., #401
Toronto, Ontario
(416) 967-1414

Make Today Count (Cancer
   patients and others with life-
   threatening diseases)
101½ S. Union St.
Alexandria, VA 22314
(703) 548-9674

March of Dimes Birth Defects
   Foundation
1275 Mamaroneck Ave.
White Plains, NY 10605
(914) 428-7100

March of Dimes (Ontario)
90 Overlea
Toronto, Ontario
(416) 425-0501

Muscular Dystrophy Association
810 Seventh Ave.
New York, NY 10019
(212) 586-0808

Muscular Dystrophy Association
of Canada
150 Eglinton East
Toronto, Ontario
(416) 488-0030

National Association for the Deaf
814 Thayer Ave.
Silver Spring, MD 20910
(301) 587-1788

Canadian Hearing Society
271 Spadina Road
Toronto, Ontario
(416) 964-9595

National Association for Visually
Handicapped
22 W 21st St.
New York, NY 10010
(212) 889-3141

National Association of Social
Workers
7981 Eastern Ave.
Silver Spring, MD 20910
(301) 565-0333

National Foundation for Asthma
P.O. Box 30069
Tucson, AZ 85751
(602) 323-6046

Asthma Society of Canada
P.O. Box 213, Station K
Toronto, Ontario
(416) 977-9684

National Foundation for Ileitis
and Colitis (Gastroenterology)
444 Park Ave., S
New York, NY 10016
(212) 685-3440

National Hemophilia Foundation
110 Green St., Rm. 406
New York, NY 10012
(212) 216-8180

Canadian Hemophilia Society
1643 Yonge Street
Toronto, Ontario
(416) 488-2244

National Homecaring Council
(Home Care)
519 C St. NE
Washington, DC 20002
(202) 547-6586

Victorian Order of Nurses
(Ontario)
76 St. Clair Ave. W.
Toronto, Ontario
(416) 928-9333

National Hospice Organization
1901 N. Ft. Myer Dr., Suite 307
Arlington, VA 22209
(703) 243-5900

The Palliative Care Foundation
33 Prince Arthur
Toronto, Ontario
(416) 922-1281

National Institute of Neurological
  and Communicative Disorders
  and Stroke
Office of Scientific and Health
  Reports
Bldg. 31, Rm. 8A-06
National Institutes of Health
Bethesda, MD 20205
(301) 496-4000

National Kidney Foundation
2 Park Ave.
New York, NY 10003
(212) 889-2210

Kidney Foundation of Canada
1300 Yonge Street
Toronto, Ontario
(416) 925-2836

National Mental Health
  Association
1021 Prince St.
Alexandria, VA 22314
(703) 684-7722

National Multiple Sclerosis
  Society
205 E. 42nd St.
New York, NY 10017
1-800-624-8236

Multiple Sclerosis Society of
  Canada
250 Bloor Street E.
Toronto, Ontario
(416) 922-6065

National Psoriasis Foundation
  (Dermatology)
6443 S.W. Beaverton Hwy.,
  Suite 210
Portland, OR 97221
(503) 297-1545

Psoriasis Education and Research
  Center
60 Grosvenor
Toronto, Ontario
(416) 964-0247

National Spinal Cord Injury
  Association
600 W. Cummings Park,
  Suite 2000
Woburn, MA 01801
(617) 935-2722

(See Canadian Paraplegic Assn.)

National Spinal Cord Injury
  Hotline
22 South Greene St.
Baltimore, MD 21201
(800) 526-3456

National Stroke Association
1420 Ogden St.
Denver, CO 80218
(303) 839-1992

(See Canadian Heart Foundation.)

Office of Cancer Communication
National Cancer Institute
Bethesda, MD 20205
(301) 496-4000

(See Natl. Cancer Institute of
  Canada.)

Paralyzed Veterans Association
801 18th St., NW
Washington, DC 20006
(202) 872-1300

(See Canadian Paraplegic Assn.)

Retinitis Pigmentosa Foundation
  Fighting Blindness
1401 Mt. Royal Ave., 4th fl.
Baltimore, MD 21217
(301) 225-9400

Society of Advancement of Travel
  for the Handicapped
26 Court St.
Brooklyn, NY 11242
(718) 858-5486

Spina Bifida Association of
  America
700 Rockville Pike, Suite 540
Rockville, MD 20852
(301) 770-7222

Spina Bifida and Hydrocephalus
  Association
55 Queen Street East
Toronto, Ontario
(416) 364-1871

Spinal Cord Society (Spinal
  Injury)
2410 Lakeview Dr.
Fergus Falls, MN 56537
(301) 739-5252

(See Canadian Paraplegic Assn.)

Stroke Club International
805 12th St.
Galveston, TX 77550
(409) 762-1022

(See Canadian Heart Association.)

Stroke Foundation Inc.
898 Park Ave.
New York, NY 10021
(212) 734-3461

(See Canadian Heart Association.)

United Cerebral Palsy
  Associations
66 E 34th St.
New York, NY 10016
(212) 947-5770

Canadian Cerebral Palsy
  Association
55 Bloor Street E.
Toronto, Ontario
(416) 923-2932

United Ostomy Association, Inc.
36 Executive Park, Suite 120
Irvine, CA 92714
(714) 660-8624

Visiting Nurse Association of
  America
518 17th St., No. 388
Denver, CO 80202
(303) 629-8622

(See Victorian Order of Nurses.)

Appendix 2

The following books are either mentioned in the text as useful resources or are publications we feel would be helpful to persons with particular illnesses. Some of these references contain guides to locate supplies, equipment, magazines, and names and addresses of a variety of illnesses or disability-related groups and organizations. These are marked with an asterisk.*

Arthritis Foundation. *Arthritis: Living and Loving: Information about Sex.* Atlanta, GA: Arthritis Foundation, 1982.

Barish, Frances. *Frommer's A Guide For the Disabled Traveler.** New York: Frommer Pasmantier, 1984. This book contains information about accessibility in hotels, restaurants, theaters, tourist sites, and transportation terminals in the United States, Canada, and Europe.

Carper, Jean. *Health Care USA.** New York: Prentice-Hall Press, 1987. Can be found in the reference section of the library. Includes lists of names, addresses, and phone numbers for doctors, hospitals, clinics, research centers, professional medical associations, self-help organizations, hospices, alternative treatments, government health agencies, publication, hotlines.

Corbet, Barry, ed. *National Resource Directory.** Massachusetts: National Spinal Cord Injury Association, 1985. This directory is an excellent information guide to services, programs, products, and equipment for all persons needing assistance whether from a disability or because of illness. It is available from the National Spinal Cord Injury Association, 149 California St., Newton, Mass. 02158. (617) 964-0521.

Corbet, Barry. *Options: Spinal Cord Injury and the Future.* Denver: A.B. Herschfeld Press, 1986. The companion for the film "Outside," *Options* provides profiles of men and women who have faced disability and worked to overcome the obstacles both emotional and physical. Although primarily about spinal injury, this film and book are excellent for the able-bodied family and friends as well as those who have paralytic problems or loss of limb.

BUILDING A NEW DREAM

Isaacs, Sally S., ed. *Community Health & Medical Guide.** New York: Health & Medical Guides, Inc., 1987–1988. A comprehensive resource book of health and medical services in Westchester County, New York. Your community library should have similar guides pertaining to your local community.

Mace, Nancy L., and Rabins, Peter V. *The 36-Hour Day.** Maryland: Warner Books, 1981. A family guide to caring for persons with Alzheimer's Disease and related dementing illnesses. Gives very useful suggestions for managing the difficult behaviors of the ill person and help with practical and emotional concerns. Also includes books, products, and organizations which can be helpful to the caretakers and family.

Maddox, Sam, ed. *Spinal Network.** Colorado: Spinal Network and Sam Maddox, 1987. A resource journal including resource connections for both the United States and Canada; contains interviews and articles on a variety of topics including medical, media and images, feature pages, sports and recreation, travel, sex and romance, legal and financial, computers, and disability rights.

Maurer, Janet R. *How to Talk to Your Doctor.* New York: Simon & Schuster, Inc., 1986. Gives information about establishing a good ongoing relationship with the doctor, and outlines the type of information you should know about your illness, medications, tests. Also discusses second opinions, specialist consultations, and when to change doctors.

Medical and Health Information Directory, 1st Edition. Can be found in the reference section of the library. This directory includes national and international associations, organizations with health-related interests, state and regional associations, federal government agencies, hospitals, health-care delivery agencies, journals, newsletters, audiovisual services, libraries, and information centers.

Minden, Sarah L. and Frankel, Debra. *Plaintalk.* New York: National Multiple Sclerosis Society, 1987. There are many publications like this one about Multiple Sclerosis for family members and the ill person available from the National MS Society or local MS Society chapters. For example:
> *Emotional Aspects of MS* by Floyd A. Davis, MD et al., National MS Society.
> *Maximizing Your Health: A Program of Graded Exercises & Meditation for Persons with Multiple Sclerosis,* edited by Robert Buxbaum, MD and Debra Frankel, MS, OTR, National MS Society.
> *Sexuality & Multiple Sclerosis* by Michael Barrett, PhD, MS Society of Canada.

Mooney, Thomas O., Theodore M. Cole, and Richard A. Chilgren. *Sexual Options for Paraplegics and Quadriplegics.* Boston: Little, Brown and Company, 1975. Gives specific and explicit (through pictures) suggestions for positions for sexual activity when mobility of arms or legs is impaired. Helpful for any ill or disabled persons regardless of cause of mobility problems who need to find alternative ways to enjoy sex or who need suggestions because of the need to make special preparation before engaging in sexual activities.

National Cancer Institute. *Taking Time.* (Bethesda Maryland) U.S. Department of Health and Human Services, National Institutes of Health. NIH Publication No. 85-2059, 1985. One of many public health pamphlets provided by the National Institutes of Health to provide support, information, and ways to cope for people with cancer and their families. Included is a guide to information services, resources, support, and service organizations.

Pitzele, Sefra Kobrin. *We Are Not Alone: Learning To Live With Chronic Illness.* Workman paperback, 1989.
Register, Cheri. *Living with Chronic Illness: Days of Patience and Passion.* Free Press, 1989.
These two books were written by women suffering from chronic illness. It is written for those who are also chronically ill to offer suggestions about how to manage their lives and their medical needs.

Schover, Leslie R. and Soren Buus Jensen. *Sexuality and Chronic Illness.* New York: The Guilford Press, 1988. Actually meant for professionals, specifically providers of sexual health care. There are good references, summary charts of the major emotional issues and physiological problems, and research studies for those who are used to academic work.

Strong, Maggie. *Mainstay.* Boston: Little, Brown & Company, 1989. Written by a spouse of a chronically ill person for spouses, to illustrate the problems and concerns and to make suggestions.

Index

Academy of Certified Social
Workers (A.C.S.W.), 58
Accident, motorcycle, case history of, 76–78
Accommodations, making, to illness or disability, 272–278,
282
Adolescents
impact of illness or disability of
parent on, 124–125, 129, 228–
233
and social isolation, case history of Hodgkin's disease in,
268–270
See also Children
Adultery, 181
AIDS, 2, 281
case history of, 90–91
and social isolation, case history of, 242, 264–268
Alcohol, medications and, 31, 33
Allergies, drug, 29–30, 33, 47
Alone, fear of being, 195
and seizures, case history of,
198–201
Alzheimer Association, 75, 139
Alzheimer's disease, 89
case history of, 72–76
and personality change, case
history of, 130, 136–140
and social isolation, case history of, 242–245, 247–250
Alzheimer's Disease and Related
Disorders Association, 139
Alzheimer Society, 75, 139

American Cancer Association, 92
American Diabetes Association,
152, 261
American Heart Association, 134,
261–262
American Lung Association, 125,
152, 248
American Medical Association,
58
American Psychological Association, 58
American Red Cross, 158, 266
Amputation, 89, 262, 277
case history of, 76, 77–78
Amyotrophic lateral sclerosis
(Lou Gehrig's disease), 53–
54, 254
Anesthesia, risk of death from,
29, 32
Anger
dealing with feelings of, 115,
279–280
against dementing illness, 243–
244
Angina pectoris, 112, 114
Antibiotics, 26, 30
Anxiety
management, products for, 61
relaxation training techniques to
reduce, 197–198
about specialist consultation, 38
symptoms related to, 23
about tests, 36
Apathy, 95, 138
vs. depression, 82

for Hodgkin's disease, 268
and relaxation training, 132
Children
    dealing with, in honest manner,
        280–281
    illness in, and emotional ex-
        haustion, 147–152
    reactions of, to illness or dis-
        ability, 70–72, 79, 107–112,
        125–127, 238–239, 240
    See also Adolescents
Chilgren, Richard A., 186, 189
Cholesterol, high, 54
Clinical social worker, 58, 59
Cole, Theodore M., 186, 189
Colitis, 2
    See also Inflammatory bowel
        disease
Colostomy, 190, 191, 192
Communication
    destructive effects of silent
        treatment on, 188–189, 193
    parent-child, about ill parent at-
        tending life event, 230–231
    "ten-minute" exercise for, 182,
        188, 193
*Community Health and Medical
    Guide*, 51, 56
Community resources, *see* Coun-
    seling; Health-care profes-
    sionals; Vocational rehabilita-
    tion services
Confidentiality, patient's right to,
    14
Consultation, *see* Specialist con-
    sultation
Control over illness, feelings of,
    104, 105, 150
Corbet, Barry, 61, 218, 272
Coronary artery bypass surgery,
    92
Coronary artery disease, medica-
    tions for, 179
Corticosteroids, 30

Counseling, 24, 56, 57, 61
    clinical social worker, 58, 59
    criteria for selecting appropri-
        ate, 59–60
    locating, 58–59, 61–62
    pastoral counselor, 58, 59
    psychiatrist, 58, 59
    psychologist, 57, 59
    See also Health-care profes-
        sionals
Course of illness, information
    about, 18, 19–21
Crises, anticipating medical, 44–
    49
Cultural attitudes, toward illness,
    8, 278–279
Cyclosporine, 28
Cystic fibrosis, 148, 150, 223
Cystic Fibrosis Associations, 152

Deafness, adaptive devices for, 61
Death
    and dying, professionals dealing
        with, 57, 58, 60
    fear of, case histories of, 195–
        203
    planning for, 48, 49, 280, 281
Dementia, 73, 243
    See also Alzheimer's disease
Denial
    and Alzheimer's disease, 243
    effective, 86–87, 198
    excessive, 198
Depression
    activities to relieve, 92–93
    case histories of, 84–87, 90–91
    causes of, 83
    at certain times of year, 87–88,
        94–95
    concept of, 80
    distinguishing between mild and
        severe, 80–81, 88
    and family resources, 93, 94
    vs. grief, 81–84, 88, 94, 280–281

Household help, hiring, 102, 125, 139, 164
Huntington's disease, 242–243
Hydrotherapy, 32
Hypertension, *see* Blood pressure, high

"I" statements, 181–182, 193
Idiopathic disease, 19
Ileostomy, sexual activity and, 186
Imagery techniques, 132
Independence
    in life-style, conflicts over maintaining, 169–172
    regaining, after illness, 144, 162
Inflammatory bowel disease, and maintaining intimacy, case history of, 174–175, 190–193
Information
    about illness, 7, 9–12, 18–21, 76, 90
    about tests, 34–35, 36, 42
Informed consent, written, 36
In-laws, difficulties with, 155–158, 165–168
Insulin injections, 150, 175, 223
Intimacy, maintaining, 174–175, 193–194
    and case history of diabetes mellitus, 175–178
    and case history of heart attack, 178–182
    and case history of inflammatory bowel disease, 190–193
    and case history of spinal-cord injury, 182–190
Isolation, fighting social, 241–242, 270–271, 277
    and AIDS, case history of, 264–268
    and Alzheimer's disease, case history of, 242–245, 247–250

and Bell's palsy, case history of, 253–261
and emphysema, case history of, 245–247, 248–250
and Hodgkin's disease, case history of, 268–270
and multiple sclerosis, case history of, 251–253
and paralysis, case history of, 261–264

Jensen, Soren Buus, 175, 189
Job(s)
    retraining, 222, 225
    supplementary, for spouse and older children, 214–215

Kaposi's sarcoma, 264
Kidney disease, 2
Kidney failure, 223

Labor, U.S. Department of, 51
Laryngectomy, 92
Life events, planning to attend, by ill or disabled, 228–233, 240
Life-style, medications and, 27
Life support systems, artificial, 48, 280
Limitations, acknowledging, 233–234, 235
Liver cirrhosis, 2
Living will, 48, 138, 280
Lou Gehrig's disease (amyotrophic lateral sclerosis), 53–54, 254
Lung diseases, 29, 31
    and meeting family social responsibilities, case history of, 227, 236–237
    See also Emphysema

Mace, Nancy L., 139
Maddox, Sam, 262

Wheelchair, 217, 221, 228, 231, 252, 256
   adaptations for, 218
   negative feelings about, 189, 190, 230
   repair service, 262
   sexual activity and, 186
   sports, 277
   and traveling, 250
Wheel Trans program (Toronto), 61
Wills
   drawing up, 280, 281
   living, 48, 138, 280
Withdrawal, 138
Work, handling changes at, 207–208, 225–226

   and case history of diabetes mellitus, 223–225
   and case history of heart attack, 208–217
   and case history of occupational asthma, 221–222
   and case history of paralysis, 217–221
Workmen's Compensation Second Injury law, 217

X rays, 35

Yeast infections, 29